COMMUNITY CARE

HC

2ND EDITION

Understanding Community Care

A Guide for Social Workers

Ann McDonald

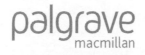

First edition 1999
Reprinted twice
Second edition 2006

Published by
PALGRAVE MACMILLAN
Houndmills, Basingstoke, Hampshire RG21 6XS and
175 Fifth Avenue, New York, N.Y. 10010
Companies and representatives throughout the world

PALGRAVE MACMILLAN is the global academic imprint of the Palgrave Macmillan division of St. Martin's Press, LLC and of Palgrave Macmillan Ltd. Macmillan is a registered trademark in the United States, United Kingdom and other countries. Palgrave is a registered trademark in the European Union and other countries.

ISBN-13: 978–1–4039–1218–3
ISBN-10: 1–4039–1218–1

This book is printed on paper suitable for recycling and made from fully managed and sustained forest sources.

A catalogue record for this book is available from the British Library.

10   9   8   7   6   5   4   3   2   1
15   14   13   12   11   10   09   08   07   06

Printed in China

To Felicity, with love

Contents

Preface to the Second Edition

This second edition of *Understanding Community Care* was prompted by the considerable developments that have taken place in legislation, policy and practice since the first edition in 1999. Social work training has undergone a significant change, with the Central Council for Education and Training in Social Work (CCETSW) being replaced by the General Social Care Council (GSCC) and the introduction of the new degree qualifications in social work. Assessment of practice competence now takes place against *National Occupational Standards for Social Work* (TOPSS, 2002), which designate key roles, and in the context of the GSCC's (2002) *Code of Practice for Social Care Workers* and the protection of the title of 'social worker'.

The substantive focus of the first edition remains, insofar as the history of community care is described and explained and is set against parallel changes in other systems such as health, education, housing and the benefits system. The retreat of the state from directly provided services has continued, but in the context of partnership and the creation of new arm's-length regulatory regimes for quality control. Research into practice confirms the development of managerialism in the organisation of formal agencies and the continuing validity of the debate as to whether or not social work is of continuing relevance within a framework of care management.

The division of material into chapters in this edition follows the same layout as the first edition, but there is a larger number of case studies and opportunities to pause and reflect, which are now located at the end of each chapter. Suggestions for further reading have been given. Links between chapters have also been made more explicit to emphasise the holistic nature of contemporary community care practice.

Acknowledgements

I would like to acknowledge, with thanks, the encouragement and help that I have continued to receive from colleagues in the School of Social Work and Psychosocial Sciences at the University of East Anglia, Norwich. Many friends, colleagues, practice teachers and students on the Dip.SW programme at UEA again have contributed ideas and practical examples of their experiences of community care. In addition, my thanks go to colleagues at Lincolnshire Partnership NHS Trust. I would particularly like to thank Kay Barker (Shail) and Bill Wivell for their interest and support throughout the writing of the first edition of *Understanding Community Care* which extended into the writing of the current edition. Undertaking such a substantial piece of work and seeing it through to its conclusion would have been impossible without the computer skills of Denys McDonald. Finally, I would like to thank my editor Catherine Gray for her encouragement and persistence.

Abbreviations

BMA	British Medical Association
CA 1989	Children Act 1989
CHAI	Commission for Healthcare Audit and Inspection
CMHNs	community mental health nurses
CMHTs	community mental health teams
CPA	care programme approach
CSCI	Commission for Social Care Inspection
DHSS	Department of Health and Social Security
Dip.SW	Diploma in Social Work
DoH	Department of Health
DSS	Department of Social Security
DWP	Department for Work and Pensions
FACS	Fair Access to Care Services
GMS	general medical services
GSCC	General Social Care Council
HiMP	health improvement and modernisation plan
HSE	Health and Safety Executive
JIP	joint investment plans
LEA	local education authority
NACRO	National Association for Care and Resettlement of Offenders
NASS	National Asylum Support Service
NHSCCA 1990	National Health Service and Community Care Act 1990
NICE	National Institute for Clinical Excellence
NISW	National Institute for Social Work
NSF	National Service Framework
PCTs	primary care trusts
PSSRU	Personal Social Services Research Unit
SCIE	Social Care Institute for Excellence
SEN	special educational needs
SSDs	social services departments
SSI	Social Services Inspectorate

Introduction

Although the National Health Service and Community Care Act (NHSCCA) 1990 is rightly seen as a watershed in the reorganisation of the delivery of services, the effect of such changes on professional development are only just beginning to be evaluated. Not for nothing was the 1989 White Paper (DoH, 1989b) subtitled *Community Care in the Next Decade and Beyond*. Systems, organisations and professions take time to adapt to fundamental changes in philosophy about how services should be delivered, to whom and at what cost. This book is intended as a guide for social workers, particularly student social workers, who are located within the system of community care. It seeks to give a realistic but hopefully positive view of the demands that are made on them by new ways of working, but also looks at opportunities for rethinking the knowledge base of social work, its skills and values, in ways appropriate to an era of change.

The historical development of community care is traced in Chapter 2, and has been well documented elsewhere (Bornat et al., 1993; Malin, 1994). Historically, there have been two separate strands of policy development; the one top down and the other bottom up, which are brought together into one system of community care. The first development was the movement to close the large institutions which had housed patients who were chronically mentally ill or had learning disabilities. This top-down strand of social policy was formalised in 1962, which means that it began more than a generation ago. Discharged patients were then to be recipients of 'care in the community'. The development of bottom-up policies designed primarily to retain people in the community and prevent, or at least delay, their movement into residential or hospital care came in the mid-1980s and was given the name 'community care'. The provision of aftercare services for people discharged from psychiatric hospital care is included in this definition, given that hospitalisation is now likely to be a temporary episode within an individual's history. Simply retaining someone in the community is no longer seen as sufficient; developing a community presence and providing care that is person-centred reflect a more recent reworking of the meaning of community care. In this way, care in the community can more properly be seen as care *by* the community and an important indicator of social inclusion. Theory and practice have together created new understandings of the meaning of the term 'community care'. Underlying these changes have been considerable debates about the proper role of the state and the rights and duties of individuals who are or may be in need of community care services. The changing role of social work in response to structural changes is a major theme explored in this book, as is the development of interagency and multidisciplinary working.

Historically, the NHSCCA 1990 was the creation of the New Right Conservative government, and reflected its commitment to principles of personal responsibility and a view of the state not as a direct provider of services but as an 'enabler'. A new language was developed, based on economic concepts, to describe the split between purchasers of services and providers of services. Social work practitioners usually found themselves on the purchaser side of this purchaser/provider split, whilst the independent sector, that is, the voluntary and private sector, was encouraged to develop as a provider of domiciliary and especially residential care. In terms of methods of working, care management became the predominant model, overshadowing person-centred approaches and arguably changing the nature of social work itself. A reliance on market mechanisms to provide the quantity and quality of care that was needed was not confined to social care but extended to healthcare, education and housing; all these services developed internal markets based on commercial principles. Individual practitioners and their managers had to develop skills in commissioning services from provider agencies, contract compliance and assessing charges, as the distinction between money and the care that it would buy became fudged.

People in receipt of such services were no longer viewed as 'clients' – a word with connotations of passivity, even dependency – but as consumers, or service users. Not only could service users complain about the quality of service they received, they also began to exert a voice in the design and evaluation of services. At the same time, informal carers were pressing for legal recognition and services in their own right, since they were providing the bulk of care in the community. Throughout this book, we explore how the service user and carer movements have challenged the historic power of professionals to decide what 'need' is and to choose how that need should be met. Because the resources devoted to community care were insufficient to meet all these different demands, difficult questions of rationing and targeting were raised. The context in which these issues were debated, however, reflected familiar social work themes of care and control, risk assessment and protection, and the empowerment of marginalised groups. A commitment to anti-discriminatory and anti-oppressive practice meant that it was particularly difficult for social work to move away from notions of universal entitlement, in recognition of the structural issues that impact on disadvantage and exclusion, to an acceptance of the use of eligibility criteria in decision-making.

The individual chapters of this book explore these debates about user empowerment and professional resilience in the context of changed organisational structures and methods of working. Chapter 1 explores the social policy background to social work in community care and the definition of the social work task in terms of care management processes. The legal framework is explored and the National Occupational Standards for social work are introduced as part of a preliminary discussion of the different functions of knowledge, skills and values. The history of community care is explored in Chapter 2 to explain 'how we got to where we are now', looking at the ideological, economic and evidence-based roots of community care as a system. Chapters 3, 4 and 5 look at the different stages of care management from assessment and care planning to monitoring and review. The question of whose definition of quality is being assessed is debated in Chapter 6, which explores the contested nature of quality assurance and quality control mechanisms. For beginning social workers, changing roles and changing values are core challenges to professionalism within community care and these are explored in Chapters 7 and 8 respectively. Chapter 9 explores and clarifies social workers' responsibilities in relation to financial matters and contains a basic overview of welfare rights. Social and healthcare needs are described in Chapter 10, which looks at the boundaries between the two systems, with particular reference to hospital discharge arrangements, the mental health system and the role of social workers in a healthcare setting. Chapter 11 looks at the contribution that good quality housing, including residential provision, can make to community care. Because community care policy and practice has developed somewhat differently for different user groups, Chapter 12 presents an overview of services for older people, people with disabilities, mental health services and other specialisms within adult care.

Community care is not a static system and although the basic core framework has proved remarkably resilient, the modernising agenda of New Labour has had an impact both on interagency working and policy development. National policy guidance has introduced standards against which local services can be measured. So, for example, National Service Frameworks (NSFs) for older people and mental health set out expectations of who should be able to access services, what types of services should be provided and the values on which services should be based. Local inequalities in charging for services have also been subject to fairer charging policy guidance, and local eligibility criteria must now conform to a national framework for distinguishing different levels of need. New forms of service delivery have also been promoted, such as the expansion of direct payments to enable individuals to purchase their own care, the separating out of housing needs from community support within the *Supporting People* programme and the introduction of intermediate care to provide rehabilitation at a stage between hospital and home. The continuing emphasis on personal responsibility is seen in the emphasis given to equality of opportunity rather than rights of citizenship in the reform of the benefits system and the targeting of scarce resources on those most in need.

Within this book, considerable emphasis is placed on legalism and due process, acknowledging the importance of a correct understanding of the legislative framework which supports community care policy and the critical nature of procedural rights where there is competition for scarce resources. Helping users of a service to understand what is available, by what means and at what cost is fundamental to a user-centred model of practice. These are principles of good administration which the system of community care is designed to uphold. This is not to imply that the care management process can or should be mechanistic; the challenge to the reflective practitioner is to integrate new models of working with skills in social casework, community work and networking. Tensions and dilemmas that may exist between economic and social objectives, between managing the budget and advocacy for the best deal possible for an individual who is seeking a service are made explicit within community care practice, at all stages of the care management process.

Finding a distinct identity for social work is a further challenge as services have been reorganised to promote interagency and multidisciplinary working. Griffiths (1988) certainly saw care management as a role which could be performed by people with backgrounds other than social work, and although some authorities have appointed only qualified social workers to assessor posts, others have recruited people from a variety of backgrounds such as nursing and allied health professions, particularly as health and social care merge into partnership arrangements or adult social services align with housing. Finding a community of knowledge and skills with social workers in childcare services is also made more complex by the development of children's trusts and proposals following the Green Paper *Every Child Matters* (DoH, 2003f) for differently skilled workers to work with children across conventional professional and organisational boundaries. The knowledge base of beginning social workers, even within the parameters of adult care, is increasingly large. Since only a minority of the population will ever come into contact with a social worker, a knowledge, for example, of mainstream services in housing, health and the social security system is obviously important. Even people with significant social needs will be catered for by mainstream services and, as ideas of normalisation and community presence take root, the numbers of vulnerable people in mainstream provision will increase. The voluntary and private sectors will also be taking large numbers of people whose needs are similar to those being maintained by the statutory sector. What service users want more than anything else is information on which to base decisions and make choices. So this book contains a considerable amount of information about what services are available, to whom and by what means of access or referrral. It is designed to enable different systems to be fitted together more smoothly by taking a holistic view of the meaning of community care services and the task of putting them together in a package of care. It seeks to explain the language of community care in a way that fits the experience of social workers and the tasks they face, with reference to underlying legislation, policy and practice guidance and recent research studies on the development of systems, roles and tasks. Although the book is aimed predominantly at a student social worker audience, it is hoped that experienced social workers and other professionals will find it a useful exposition of some basic concepts.

CHAPTER 1

Social Work within Community Care

Introduction

Although the focus of this book is the delivery of social care services in the context of community care, many of the innovations that were introduced with the National Health Service and Community Care Act (NHSCCA) 1990, such as health, education, social security, housing and criminal justice, have been paralleled in other services. The interconnectedness of such services is not a creation of community care, but the essential bedrock for the holistic assessment of need on which service delivery is based. Each of these services has experienced the growth of managerialism, the separation of purchaser from provider functions and the targeting of resources on those most in need or most at risk. Detailed consideration needs to be given to similarities and differences in the organisation and delivery of these services and their value base to understand the experience of social workers within them. Only in such a way can opportunities for, and barriers to, interdisciplinary working be highlighted.

Social policy perspectives

The social policy perspectives examined here are relevant to all adult services, for example services for older people, people with mental health problems, those with physical or learning disabilities and recipients of drug and alcohol services. Means and Smith (1994) recount the long history of neglect which is common to these groups, both in the unsatisfactory nature of institutional provision and the persistent failure to develop adequate community-based systems of support. They use the perspectives of political economy, institutions and service neglect, informal care and service neglect, and cultural stereotypes to explain both inertia in policy change and the marginalisation of these groups.

The political economy perspective focuses on changes in the mode of production and the shift from a communal agrarian economy to an urban economy based on individual waged labour. Those who were seen as unproductive – the old, the sick – were necessarily marginalised within such a system. By the provision of pension and welfare benefits they were moved into structured dependency on the state (Townsend, 1981). Minimal provision for older people, no longer valued as workers, could also be used to socialise a younger generation into the virtues of family responsibility, thrift and saving for the future (Thompson and Thompson, 1993). The current debate around funding continuing care for older people draws heavily on the political economy perspective. Ageism and disablism are thus seen as structurally entrenched in social and economic policy. The claims of these groups are not acknowledged as rights of citizenship, but are granted as privileges or concessions. Equal opportunities legislation, such as the Disability Discrimination Act 1996, is used to deflect dissent by the granting of concessions, not rights.

For people dependent on public welfare, Means and Smith (1994) identify a frequent theme in the literature on institutions: that many were designed to impose stigma on residents and serve as a warning to others. Institutions, typically in remote locations, isolated residents from the community as a whole. Institutional provision, however, is not cheap; hence the attractiveness of arrangements to support people in the community, possibly at a lower cost and certainly with greater control over access to expensive resources. There would inevitably be a difficult transitional period when institutions closed before community resources developed sufficiently to meet this new demand.

Reliance on informal care giving by family and friends is not a creation of community care policy, but a background to much service neglect in the past. Fear of undermining the family as an institution, as well as increasing public expenditure, may serve as a justification for placing limits on the availability of domiciliary care and emphasising personal and familial responsibility. This, of course, places an enormous burden on informal carers, the majority of whom are women. Reaction has come from feminist writings (Dalley, 1988; Finch, 1989) who see the exploitation of women's labour as inevitable without heavy state investment in care, including residential care. This feminist critique of community care is based on research into carers' domestic, family and work commitments. Whether it creates unhelpful divisions between disabled people who receive help and those who provide it is an issue raised by Jenny Morris (1993). The role of informal carers within community care is further discussed in Chapter 7.

Cultural stereotypes about ageing and disability have informed service provision. Negative stereotypes of old age emphasise physical and mental decline, and dependency. Old age is presented not as a developmental stage, but as a 'problem' for policy-makers to address. The Rising Tide initiative in the 1980s, with its references to a 'demographic timebomb' (Health Advisory Service, 1983; Bernard, 1987), is an example of this. Disability, conversely, has been presented in legislation and in social policy as personal tragedy in avoidance of a collective need to adapt the assumptions and arrangements of non-disabled people which act as barriers in the fields of education, housing and employment among others (Oliver, 1996). An unsympathetic legislative framework has inhibited the development of anti-discriminatory practice with this group of people.

The social policy of community care

The analysis of social policy may conveniently be presented in a social democratic, Marxist, feminist or New Right framework (Thompson and Thompson, 1993). The social democratic view is that change is incremental, based on consensus and a humanitarian reaction to objectively verifiable 'facts' such as demographic change or increased prosperity. A Marxist analysis of the same welfare provision is that it excludes unproductive people from mainstream employment or education in order to support the major aim of efficiency in production (Guillemard, 1983). The role of women is then to provide domestic services at no extra cost. The feminist perspective on 'care' similarly sees the interests of women as submerged under the demands of the other members of the family or community. Women provide free labour under such a system and enable the state to continue to play a marginal role. The emphasis on personal and family responsibility was a theme taken up by the New Right: it informs much of community care policy, particularly in its emphasis on the residual nature of public provision.

The New Right approach is not confined to the provision of social welfare services. Common themes for the delivery of public service were developed throughout the period of the last Conservative government (1979–97). These common themes were:

- the purchaser/provider split
- the mixed economy of care
- targeting
- consumerism
- quality mechanisms.

The split between purchasers and providers of services was not an innovation as such, since those functions had often been divided administratively within the same organisation. What was new was the concept of the 'enabling state', whose role was to encourage the development of service provision within the independent sector, not through direct provision. The services to be provided were not necessarily universal in character, but were to be targeted on those in greatest need. Who defines what need is, and according to what outcome measures, therefore becomes crucial. Entitlement to benefits and/or services on the basis simply of citizenship was to be further undermined by the spread of means-testing to pay for services and the notion of consumerism; greater freedom of choice for service users was an important theme together with better complaints mechanisms for those who were dissatisfied with standards of service. Concern for quality led to a greater emphasis on standard-setting and inspection, covering public as well as private provision. This greater concern with regulation was somewhat ironic, given the overall belief in the effectiveness of market forces in increasing efficiency by increasing competition in quasi-markets. A whole new language had to be learned.

The NHSCCA 1990 places a duty on local authorities to assess those who appear to be in need of community care services. A common framework is thus provided within which a range of people with different individual needs are to be assessed and have their needs met. However, within this common framework, different patterns of provision have developed and are likely to continue to develop according to age and type of disability. Some groups which have historically been marginalised, such as those with substance misuse problems, may take advantage of new administrative arrangements and ways of working to transform service provision. For other groups, such as older people, the community care changes may have led to reduced levels of provision and an obligation to pay for the care that is received. A brief overview of service developments within community care for different service user groups is given in Chapter 12.

The social work task

The Quality Assurance Agency's benchmark for social work and social policy (QAA, 2000) and the National Occupational Standards (TOPSS, 2002) for the new social work degree refer to an indicative knowledge base, the use of evidence and theoretical perspectives and specific and transferable skills. Their particular application to social work in community care will be highlighted in the ensuing chapters. Note that the emphasis is on social work practice, and not on care management. Whether or not care management has taken over from social work as the professional role within community care is discussed further in Chapter 7. Certainly, the skills and methods of social work practice are appropriate for use in a care management role (Sheppard, 1995). The skills of social work, it is argued, extend beyond this role to the provision of therapeutic interventions and support not necessarily contained within the brief of a care manager, who is seen predominantly as a commissioner of services. Yet the importance of skills to meet the psychological and emotional needs of vulnerable adults must constantly be emphasised. This is true at the point of assessment as well as subsequent stages. This means that it exists independently of the purchaser/provider split, which (artificially) seeks to separate out assessment and provider functions.

Care management is the preferred means by which the assessment of needs, planning, monitoring and review is to be carried out (DoH, 1990a). Practice guidance to the implementation of the NHSCCA 1990 is officially formulated in the *Managers' Guide* (SSI/DoH, 1991a) and the *Practitioners' Guide* (SSI/DoH, 1991). Care management as described in the *Practitioners' Guide* is a process comprising seven stages:

1   Publishing information
2   Determining the level of assessment
3   Assessing need
4   Care planning
5   Implementing the care plan
6   Monitoring
7   Reviewing.

The guidance encourages practitioners to view the process in cyclical terms, with a review of unmet need informing the assessment process, both on an individual level and in terms of planning services at the macro-level (see Figure 1.1).

Social workers will be most commonly employed within this process on the purchaser side. They also have a role within the provision of services in daycare

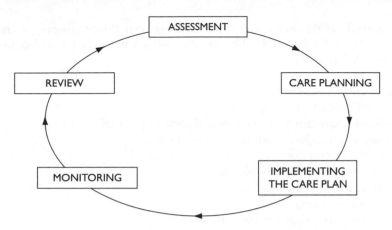

Figure 1.1 The cycle of care management

or residential units, or in specialist roles in resource teams. They will not necessarily operate in this provider role within the statutory sector. Social workers may be employed within the voluntary or private sector in any of these provider roles, or, indeed, in an assessor role, where the provision of public funding is not an issue. Any description of what social work is in community care has to take these variations into account. The dichotomy of roles within the purchaser/provider split in some ways reflects the social care planner/counsellor divide inherent in social work, set out for consideration in the Barclay Report (1982). Thus social work has always had to struggle with these two aspects of its role. Community care has not created the dichotomy, but it has emphasised it. The challenge now is to retain the dialogue between the two roles and not set up barriers, whether organisational or intellectual, which prevent the skills of one being used for the benefit of the other.

Parallels with the Children Act 1989

Change within childcare services during this same period was driven by a desire for a clear and more efficient legal framework as well as a professional desire to work in partnership, influenced by research on the importance of family life for children. The value base of the Children Act (CA) 1989 is made explicit in the first of many volumes of guidance on the Act, *The Care of Children: Principles and Practice in Regulations and Guidance* (DoH, 1989a). The values on which the guidance is based are those of respect for individual needs and potential, the development of working partnerships with parents and families and the avoidance of discrimination or stigma. This officially sanctioned and professionally agreed value base was absent from community care legislation, even though there are similarities in structure and concerns between childcare and community care legislation.

Macdonald (1991) draws useful parallels between the provisions of the CA 1989 and the NHSCCA 1990. The specific issues which are paralleled in both pieces of legislation are:

- assessments of need with regular reviews
- clear and explicit planning
- published information on services and eligibility criteria
- complaints procedures and user representation
- minimum intervention
- practical support to carers/parents
- service agreements and charges
- interagency working
- provision of day/respite/preventive services
- registers of potential users
- registration and inspection
- quality control and quality assurance.

Some authorities have also adopted a care management role within children's services. Benefits have been perceived to be that work is more clearly focused and time-limited, there is a stronger emphasis on outcomes and the development of provider services in the independent sector is more clearly emphasised. Care management as a method can thus span organisational divisions, and recent developments in children's services – the creation of children's trusts, an NSF (DoH, 2004b) and a shared assessment framework – parallel earlier developments in adult services.

The legal framework of community care

The NHSCCA 1990 does not offer a comprehensive legislative framework for the practice of social work in adult care. In this it differs from the CA 1989 which, with the exception of adoption, replaces previous legislation and applies the same principles to voluntary and compulsory intervention. The legislative framework for working with adults cannot be understood from a reading of the NHSCCA alone; reference needs to be made to previous legislation relevant to the provision of services, and important pieces of legislation on disability and mental health are to be found outside the framework of the Act. Lewis and Glennerster (1996) see the history of the NHSCCA as almost wholly driven by financial considerations, in particular by the need to redress the 'perverse incentive' for the growth of the adult residential sector which was based on unlimited access to social security funding. Devolving gatekeeping powers to local authorities gave them lead agency status in the provision of services in the community; nevertheless, the limits of their discretion could be controlled by central government through the funding process. Allocation of these scarce resources could therefore proceed on the basis of 'need', with the professionals as intermediaries in defining and assessing need. It would still be possible, under this sort of regime, for the state to act as a 'facilitator and enabler', but this would be far from a policy of open access to services. The fundamentals of the community care system such as the purchaser/

provider split and care management are, however, not statutory, they are a creation of policy and practice. The absence of legal imperatives has meant that the pattern and pace of change has been different in different parts of the country; different models of care management have been developed to meet different organisational objectives and also different views on, for example, professional autonomy and user involvement.

It is paradoxical that such uncertainties should have existed within an administrative system which emphasises legalism. Quality assurance – building quality into systems through the registration of services and by inspection and review – is based on an assumption that there is a common agreement on standards and objective ways of measuring them. Legalism, however, does not necessarily extend to support for entitlement to services as a matter of legal right. There may be an expressed duty on social services departments (SSDs) to provide services of a particular sort such as domiciliary or residential care, but access to such services is expressed in terms of need, not in terms of universal entitlement. Nor does legislation specify how much of a certain type of benefit should be made available to meet the demands placed on it; it may be very little, or it may be a good deal. Much emphasis is then placed on devising procedures for a 'fair' allocation of services and a due process model for dealing with potential disputes. Local authorities will devise procedures manuals for their staff to seek to encourage conformity with this due process model, and will reserve some decisions with greater-than-average resource implications to senior managers to deal with strategically.

Clients, service users and consumers

The public relations task of making potential users aware of what services are available and how they can be accessed is crucial to a consensual model of practice. Despite official encouragement to focus on ways of disseminating information, the evidence has been that local authorities are not good at letting people know what services are available (Age Concern, 1994; Mencap, 1995). At practitioner level, an exchange model of assessment, which sees the potential user as at least an equal partner in the process of assessing needs, is dependent on that person having sufficient knowledge and information about what is available in order to make an informed choice (Smale and Tuson, 1993). A new use of language has emerged which in itself changes expectations of roles. The trend is away from the use of the term 'client' (which implies a passive recipient of a professionally determined service) towards the term 'service user' or 'consumer', which connotes a more active and discriminating role. As service users are increasingly likely to be contributing financially to the cost of the services they receive, they will seek wider choice and value for money in the services on offer.

Whilst consumer sovereignty may be in the ascendancy for those people who are able to exercise choice, there is, at the same time, a dilemma for social workers in community care in balancing the rights of vulnerable, and often very ill, people against pressure from the wider society to deal with threats to safety and public order. This is most clearly manifest in social work with people who are mentally ill, where recently there has been rapid legislative change designed to secure greater monitoring of, and control over, people in the community. There are similar dilemmas in work with people who are vulnerable to exploitation by others, or at risk of self-neglect in the community, and who may lack the mental capacity to consent to the provision of services designed for their protection. Fundamental issues of citizenship and civil rights are at stake here, and the claims of social work to speak for those who are oppressed or marginalised in society are being put to the test (Jordan, 1996). Issues of anti-oppressive and anti-discriminatory practice often focus in practice on risk assessment and risk management in work in adult services. Community care can therefore never be seen as the atheoretical application of services to willing and informed consumers.

Knowledge, skills and values

The relationship between theory and practice hinges on the question 'How do knowledge and thought influence or inform our actions?' (Thompson, 1995). But this combination of knowledge and action is insufficient without the integration of social work values. Formal knowledge may come from the social sciences, psychology or an understanding of legislation; practice will give us experience in observation and application. Reflection and analysis link theory and practice, so that by the application of theory we can better understand why we do what we do at more than an intuitive or learning-by-rote level. This process, which leads on to hypothesis-testing and new forms of experimentation, does not end with the emergence of the 'reflective practitioner'. The process is more likely to be a cyclical one, in an attempt to bridge the gap between 'the high ground of academic rigour and the swampy lowlands of practice' (Schön, 1993).

Payne (2002) emphasises the importance of reflexivity in social work, in the sense of gaining evidence about the consequences and effectiveness of our actions which in turn modifies our approach to practice in the future. This approach to the production and nurturing of a reflective practitioner is the aim of any professional training. The ability to integrate values into practice means that social work students must identify and question their own values and prejudices and their implications for practice. The complexities of this sort of exhortation at both a theoretical and practical level are discussed in Chapter 8.

The functions of social work

What is the function of social work within this system of community care? Is it there to serve the system or ameliorate it? This is, of course, not a new debate. Social work has never resolved the dilemma of whether it is a service to the state in the pursuit of social policy through the enforcement of legislation and the rationing of scarce resources, or a means by which marginalised and disadvantaged groups can have their needs drawn to the attention of service providers. The professional identity of the social worker in adult care is also subject to challenges, both external and internal.

The role of the care manager is one open to people from a variety of backgrounds, not explicitly limited to social work. In the National Occupational

Standards, no distinction is drawn between the key skills required in childcare and adult care and evidence of competence is based holistically on work with individuals, families, carers, groups and communities; a unity of interests across the profession is assumed and the transferability of skills is sought. To what extent is the development of community care as an administrative system a threat to the profession of social work? The threat may be twofold. Firstly, the core feature of a profession is the possession of a distinctive body of knowledge and skills: if other types of people can become care managers, where does this leave social work? Secondly, the growth of managerialism may pose a threat to the autonomy of social workers, insofar as a narrow administrative definition of tasks may reduce the scope for professional discretion.

A rigid purchaser/provider split may give rise to an administrative model of care management, whereby traditional social work skills such as counselling are labelled as the prerogative of providers and are squeezed out (Lewis and Glennerster, 1996). This is despite Challis's early assertion (1992) that social work skills are important within the care management process, in engaging the client, forming a relationship and giving advice. Petch (1996) perceives a distinction between role and task. Care management may be the job description of individuals appointed as care managers, or it may be carried out by social workers alongside other social work tasks, which include the provision of therapy. Designing, putting into place and supporting a package of care for a person in the community is not just putting together a basket of goods and services, it is the creation and management of a complex set of human relationships (Smale and Tuson, 1993). It involves skills in negotiation and planning which are based on a sound understanding of the social and psychological development of human beings. It also involves practice skills such as interviewing, communicating, assessing, recording, counselling and mobilising resources, all central skills in social work training (Coulshed and Orme, 1998). This has led Sheppard (1995) to conclude that social workers' knowledge, skills and values equip them particularly well to act as lead professionals in a care management role.

Challenges of modernisation

A change in government in 1997 led to changes in community care policy. *Modernising Social Services* (DOH, 1998a) and the *National Priorities Guidance* (DoH, 1998) set the modernising agenda of the New Labour government to construct new forms of service delivery, based on partnership rather than competition, and supplement market forces with arm's-length processes of regulation and inspection. Henwood and Waddington (2002) identify the 'modernisation imperative' as having four components:

- The driving-up of service quality through best value and the 'four Cs' – consultation, comparison, challenge and competition
- The promotion of evidence-based care
- Developing accessible and individually tailored services
- Improving partnership.

Best value requirements and performance indicators provide a national system for assessing and comparing the delivery of services locally. Commenting on the move from direct provision to market care, Means et al. (2002, p. 24) observe:

> Central government may believe in markets and competition, but it also believes that its social policy objectives can only be met through the stimulus of extensive surveillance.

Organisations such as the Social Care Institute for Excellence (SCIE) and the National Institute for Clinical Excellence (NICE) have been created to gather and disseminate best examples of evidence-based practice. The Commission for Social Care Inspection (CSCI) also works at arm's length from the providers of residential and domiciliary care, and according to National Minimum Standards to regulate formal providers. NSFs (in mental health and for older people) not only stipulate standards of service, but also promote models of service (for example assertive outreach, intermediate care) by which outcomes will be achieved. Individually tailored services are at the heart of person-centred care for people with learning difficulties within the White Paper *Valuing People* (DoH, 2000b), which also formally requires interagency cooperation through the formation of partnership boards. Concern with crude distinctions such as the purchaser/ provider split is replaced by a shift from process to content and outcomes. Henwood and Waddington (2002, para. 1.7) describe what has become known as the 'third way' as intending to:

> move the focus away from who provides the care, and place it firmly on the quality of services experienced by, and outcomes achieved for, individuals and their carers and families.

Divisions between and within organisations are thus subordinated to partnership tasks, evidenced by: the development of partnership trusts and care trusts for the delivery of health-related services; the creation of Sure Start, 'extended' schools and the Connexions service to provide a bridge between education and social care; and the development of the New Deal providing back-to-employment support for those on benefits.

Outcomes themselves are disaggregated into three different types of achievement (Henwood and Waddington, 2002), each measurable qualitatively as well as quantitatively:

- *Maintenance outcomes* – based on quality of life measures such as cleanliness and security, but also social participation and control
- *Change outcomes* – tackling barriers to achieve quality of life or reducing risks, for example improving relationships, assisting recovery and rehabilitation
- *Process outcomes* – looking at the impact of the way in which the package of services is delivered against measures such as cultural sensitivity, choice and respect.

The emphasis has thus shifted from the mechanics of maintaining people in the community to tackling social exclusion and increasing participation, as well as increasing individual choice.

Research commissioned by the Joseph Rowntree Foundation as part of the Shaping our Lives project reviewed principles as well as practice in consultation (Turner, 2003). Taking a collectivist view, respondents believed that access to services, including housing, education, employment and transport, as well as health, social care and benefits should be seen as a basic human right. National standards on involvement were sought to prevent consultation from being meaningless and ensure that national strategies across services were developed. This emphasis on the democratisation of services from the grassroots as a political value is at odds with other values within the regulatory system. In a study of joint reviews, Humphrey (2003, p. 16) discerns four sets of values referred to in New Labour, Audit Commission and Joint Review texts to justify the regulatory apparatus put in place around best value:

1   *Economic values* around economy, efficiency and cost-effectiveness
2   *Scientific values* around facts and evidence (performance indicator statistics, for example) that help to assure us of the independent status and impartial stance of the regulators
3   *Political values* around democracy – the regulators consult with a variety of local stakeholders and their reports are a vehicle for promoting the public accountability of public authorities
4   *Welfare values*, which may be collective (inclusivity and community) or individual (the right to exercise choice and register complaints).

Regulatory agencies are observed to be struggling in practice with tradeoffs between: statistics and substance; cost and quality; and minority and majority needs. The final tradeoff is particularly important to social work, operating as it does with those who are marginalised by society, but in a context in which 'public services will be assessed in accordance with how far they can propel people into the majority camp' (Humphrey, 2003, p. 19). Social work as a profession exists because of contradictions to one of the basic tenets of *Modernising Social Services* (DoH, 1998a) that the provision of welfare services can be seen in universalist terms rather than as a system which deals with social casualties.

Models of practice

While theories, both political and economic, may explain why new organisational systems emerge, and how inputs can be related to outcomes in terms of increasing welfare, the real focus of our interest is what happens on the ground. Social work in community care has evolved important new models of practice. There are different ways of organising services, different mixes of professional expertise, for example in community mental health teams or community learning disability teams, and different approaches to user involvement in the design and delivery of services. Community care has also expanded to include new services for people with HIV/AIDS and drug or alcohol problems and has absorbed pressures from central government to respond to asylum seekers and refugees. The history of community care and an examination of the legal context within which it operates are the subject matter of Chapter 2. The legal paradigm of rights, duties, powers and remedies is an essential framework within which individual authorities' interpretation of their obligations to citizens may be judged. Chapters 7 and 8 explore the impact of community care on the changing roles and values of the social work profession. The emphasis throughout is on the practicalities of working within changing systems and seizing the opportunities for innovation that they present as well as noting their limitations.

National Occupational Standards

The National Occupational Standards for Social Work (TOPSS, 2002) set the framework for contemporary practice. They comprise six key roles, the practice components of which are broken down into units through which competence in the key roles can be evidenced. For each unit there is also an indicative knowledge base. The National Occupational Standards are set within the International Association of Schools of Social Work (IASSW, 2001) 'statement of the key purpose of social work' as:

> a profession which promotes social change, problem solving in human relationships and the empowerment and liberation of people to enhance well-being. Utilising theories of human behaviour and social systems, social work intervenes at the points where people interact with their environments. Principles of human rights and social justice are fundamental to social work.

The standards are designed to be applicable to all settings and reflect the changing context and expectations of social work practice. They try to capture the holistic approach of social workers that differentiates their role from that of other professionals with whom they work, whilst trying to ensure consistency with the standards and codes of ethics of other professional groups. The standards recognise the need for social workers to manage some inherent tensions between work focused on those requiring services, and their carers, and statutory requirements. Key roles 1–4 cover the practice of social work and are explored predominantly in Chapters 3–5 of this book, in the context of assessment, planning, monitoring and review. Key roles 5–6 refer to the social worker as an accountable and professionally competent practitioner and underpin all other activities; they are explored predominantly in Chapters 6–8 and Chapter 12.

Concluding comments

This chapter looked at changes in policy and practice as the theoretical framework of community care has developed under successive governments. The new social work degree emphasises the acquisition of skills through the key roles that all social workers undertake and links the skills to challenges encountered during the 200 days of practice learning. Despite divergences between adults' and children's services, qualification requirements seek to preserve a unity within the profession through shared knowledge, skills and values. Although Chapter 2 traces the particular history of community care, much of the language and many of the concepts that it introduces are transferable to contemporary social work within other settings and with other user groups.

PAUSE AND REFLECT

Reflect back on your reasons for wanting to become a social worker, and think about what influenced your choice of career. List the influences in order of importance to you. Some things you might consider are: the opportunity to 'make a difference'; the chance to use interpersonal skills; good role models provided by social workers you have known; employment opportunities and career structure. To what extent does the IASSW statement of the key purpose of social work match your list?

CASE STUDY

Key roles

Heather Green is aged 85 and was admitted to hospital after a stroke four weeks ago. Her condition has now stabilised and she has had some input from the occupational therapist and physiotherapist on the ward. Her consultant considers that she will be fit for discharge in two weeks' time and has asked ward staff to make a referral to the social work department at the hospital. The case is referred to you.

Identify the key roles that you would evidence in working with Mrs Green to facilitate her discharge from hospital. What further information would you need to have about her circumstances, and with whom would you liaise?

Using key roles 1–6, you might consider the following points.

■ Key role 1: Prepare for and work with individuals, families, carers, groups and communities to assess their needs and circumstances
  What are Mrs Green's needs in this situation? How will you make the first approach to her, explaining your role? Is there any interview schedule that you will be expected to follow? Does Mrs Green have a carer in the community? Are family members to be involved? What support can Mrs Green's community give? What information can other professionals give you about Mrs Green's needs and her level of fitness?

■ Key role 2: Plan, carry out, review and evaluate social work practice with individuals, families, carers, groups and communities and other professionals
  Is there any opportunity to plan Mrs Green's discharge in a multidisciplinary meeting, such as a ward round, involving Mrs Green and her family? Are there any time constraints within which you must operate? What resources are there and how appropriate are they to Mrs Green's needs? Are there eligibility criteria that have to be met? What outcome are you aiming for and how will you review and evaluate whether it has been achieved?

■ Key role 3: Support individuals to represent their needs, views and circumstances
  Does Mrs Green need assistance in putting forward her point of view? Is an independent advocate needed? Is one available? Are carers offered their own assessment, not assuming that they are willing to carry on caring, but supporting them if they wish to do so?

- Key role 4:   Manage risk to individuals, families, carers, groups, communities, self and colleagues
  Be aware that risk involves a balancing of positives as well as negatives and may be perceived differently by each of these groups. In particular, the organisation may be 'at risk' if Mrs Green's discharge is delayed and this may have repercussions for the individual worker.

- Key role 5:   Manage and be accountable, with supervision and support, for your own social work practice within your organisation
  Mrs Green will not be the only referral that you are given. How do you prioritise this work within your caseload to meet the deadline that has been set? What paperwork needs to be completed and how will you record your actions? What supervision is available to you in identifying and dealing with the relevant issues and what use will you make of other support inside and outside the agency? How much autonomy is available to you in making decisions and dealing with outside agencies, such as domiciliary care providers and residential homes, and in carrying out financial assessments?

- Key role 6:   Demonstrate professional competence in social work practice
  Are you able to understand and choose between different theories and models of social work practice with vulnerable adults? Are you up to date with legislation relating to hospital discharge and research on the impact of ageing and ill-health? Do you have problem-solving skills in gathering information, assessing its reliability and dealing with professional dilemmas? Can you evaluate ethical issues and are you aware of the impact of discrimination and the requirements of anti-oppressive practice?

FURTHER READING

Malin, N., Wilmot, S. and Manthorpe, J. (2002) *Key Concepts and Debates in Health and Social Policy.* Buckingham: Open University Press.
Explores the history of community care, clearly explains relevant concepts and examines the development of 'third way' politics in the late 1990s and beyond.

Means, R., Richards, S. and Smith, R. (2003) *Community Care: Policy and Practice* (3rd edn). Basingstoke: Palgrave Macmillan.
The third edition of what has become a classic text on the development of British social policy in community care. Includes European perspectives and a comprehensive guide to further reading.

CHAPTER 2

The History of Community Care

Introduction

This chapter examines the history of community care and its implications for social work practice. Changes in other areas of social policy are also charted in order to highlight parallel developments. The legal framework within which social welfare policies are defined and delivered is described. This change to the statutory framework inevitably has had an impact on social work, perhaps changing its very nature, insofar as social work exists as a statutorily sanctioned activity (Davies, 1994).

The impetus for change to a system of community care was not professionally driven; it came from the policies of a Conservative government committed to free-market principles and a reduction in public spending. Social work in the mid-1980s was predominantly generic, rooted in casework as a method of intervention and unconcerned with economics. Social work was largely the prerogative of statutory agencies, the effectiveness of which was not, on the whole, subject to an analysis in terms of value for money. During the latter part of the 1980s, however, there were a number of reports published which disclosed inefficiencies within the existing system and proposed changes which more transparently linked resources to outcomes. The concentration was on process rather than skills and on systems rather than human relationships. Not surprisingly, the social work position in all this was a reactive one, and social work today is still engaged in the struggle to re-establish its role in the new order which emerged. Thus some knowledge of history is fundamental to operating creatively as a social worker within the National Occupational Standards.

Community care policy in the 1980s

There were three strands to community care policy in the 1980s: the ideological, the outcomes of research and the economic. Each is now explained.

The ideological

The ideological stance was promulgated by Norman Fowler, then secretary of state for social services, in his speech in Buxton, Derbyshire in 1986, in which he talked about 'rolling back the boundaries of the state', envisaging a fundamental shift from the role of the state as provider to that of enabler. In December 1986,

Norman Fowler asked Sir Roy Griffiths, who had previously been instrumental in reviewing management in the NHS, to conduct a review of community care policy and, in particular, in his terms of reference:

> to review the way in which public funds are used to support community care policy and to advise on the options for action that would improve the use of those funds.

The Griffiths Report (1988) was prompted by two earlier reports which highlighted deficiencies and contradictions in policy. The House of Commons Select Committee Report on Community Care in 1984–5 (Social Services Committee, 1985) had been critical of the inadequate care provided to patients discharged from long-stay psychiatric hospitals into the community and the Audit Commission (1986) had drawn attention to the 'perverse incentive' provided to (mainly elderly) people to enter residential care by the direct payment of fees from the DHSS without a proper assessment of need. Griffiths (1988) recommended that local authorities should take the lead role in planning, according to local priorities, and that responsibility for funding residential care should be transferred from the DHSS to local authorities. Private enterprise and voluntary agencies would be encouraged to act as providers of care. The system would be managed for individuals through a process of case (later care) management, possibly involving a number of different professional groups.

Initially, the Griffiths Report was not well received by central government because of the greater discretion it appeared to give to local government – which could be of a different political complexion from central government. Ultimately, however, the opportunity to stem a bill for private residential care that had grown from £10 million in 1979 to £1000 million in 1989 proved irresistible, and the Griffiths recommendations were largely replicated in the 1989 White Paper *Caring for People: Community Care in the Next Decade and Beyond* (DoH, 1989b). The objectives of the White Paper were stated to be:

1. to promote the development of domiciliary, day and respite services to enable people to live in their own homes wherever feasible and sensible
2. to ensure that service providers make practical support for carers a high priority
3. to make proper assessment of need and good care management the cornerstone of high-quality care
4. to promote the development of a flourishing independent sector alongside good quality public services
5. to clarify the responsibilities of agencies and so make it easier to hold them to account for their performance
6. to secure better value for taxpayers' money by introducing a new funding structure for social care.

The outcomes of research

Research published by the Personal Social Services Research Unit (PSSRU) at the University of Kent and commissioned by the DHSS also appeared to confirm the value of targeting scarce resources on those most vulnerable to admission to expensive residential care (Davies and Challis, 1986). The research concentrated chiefly on frail elderly people, but findings derived from it were extrapolated to other user groups (Phillips, 1996). The 'production of welfare' approach adopted by the PSSRU adapted what was basically an economic model by evaluating inputs (staff time, physical resources and money) against outputs (length of time remaining in the community, improvement in carer stress). The process which most efficiently achieved these outcomes was presented as that of care management – as a system which mediates needs, resources and interpersonal relationships. Pilling (1992) usefully summarises the different projects undertaken and their major findings. The Kent project (1985–9) examined the effectiveness of care in the community for frail elderly people when managed by care managers with limited caseloads and access to community resources, including local volunteers who were paid a minimal wage. The Darlington project, by contrast, targeted potential continuing care hospital patients in order to demonstrate that care in the community could be equally cost-effective (Challis et al., 1995). Multipurpose workers were used who were able to work across the healthcare/ social care divide. The American experience of case management also highlighted the value of this method in bringing together diverse providers within a 'package of care' (Raiff and Shore, 1993). Parallel to these community care projects were 28 care in the community projects which looked at the resettlement of former long-stay patients into the community. It was a condition of funding that these projects incorporated a system of care management.

The reports subsequently produced on these early projects are, from a social work perspective, curiously unsatisfying. Care management as a system is divorced from any sense of the established social work role in settling people into communities or providing support services for them to remain there. Few examples are given of direct interventions between care managers, service users and their families, which means that the potency of skills in building relationships rather than organising resources is not visible. The health/social care divide is also presented as unproblematic when this clearly was not the case, especially in the Darlington project, where there are instances of hospital consultants readmitting patients on their own analysis of risk without consultation with the project team (Challis et al., 1995).

The economic

The development of ideas about community care in the 1980s was fundamentally based on free-market principles. This concept of the commissioning state rather than the state as direct provider was also seen in the development of new patterns in the provision of other fundamental services such as health, education and housing. Thus, for social services, the local authority would purchase services from a range of voluntary and private sector providers as well as, or instead of, making available its own in-house services such as domiciliary care or daycare. Under the health service reorganisation, health authorities and GP fundholders would purchase services from NHS hospitals and community trusts. In education, the local education authority would assess a child as having special educational needs, but might have to purchase educational services from grant-maintained schools outside the local education authority (LEA) system. Local authority housing departments were also less likely to build their own housing stock than to nominate tenants to housing associations for social housing.

In all this, certain trends are discernible:

- public sector direct provision of services is becoming the exception rather than the norm
- a multiplicity of care services are, potentially at least, able to develop
- the user of services is treated as a consumer, rather than a client
- accountability for quality of service is divided between organisations in the public and private sectors.

The mixed economy of care

The services that the purchaser/provider split creates are known as 'quasi-markets' (Le Grand and Bartlett, 1993). They are markets (in the economic sense of the term) because they replace monopolistic state providers with competitive independent suppliers. However, in contrast to conventional markets, all these organisations are not necessarily out to maximise profits. On the demand side, consumer purchasing power is not directly expressed in money terms by the ultimate user of the service. Instead, agents for the user (care managers) are the people who exercise choice and purchasing power from an agency budget set aside for that purchase. Such quasi-markets are often not based on free competition in terms of standards or quality of service; residential care, for example, remains highly regulated according to national legislation.

One of the assumptions made in the development of a mixed economy of care is that the public/private and voluntary sectors are qualitatively different from each other. Taylor et al. (1995) reject this notion by pointing out similarities as well as differences. Funding and contract arrangements meant that the interests of the statutory sector had a strong stake in the survival of many voluntary organisations. The private sector itself was also found to be diverse, ranging from small family firms and partnerships to large corporate concerns with share-holders. The independent sector had been joined by a diverse group of not-for-profit organisations, such as housing associations and floated-off trusts and companies. Taylor et al. (1995) break down these not-for-profit organisations into three groups:

- *community* – run for and by people from a particular neighbourhood or (possibly ethnic) community
- *user* – run by service users or ex-users, or by carers for carers
- *donor* – where people give their time or money to help others.

They see the most important qualitative difference as being between organisations run by and for users, and organisations run on more paternalistic lines. What distinguishes private organisations from the rest is a lack of mutuality and sense of collective empowerment, as well as an absence of a campaigning stance on behalf of service users.

The replacement of grant aid by a contract culture to fund the voluntary sector has had major effects (Russell, 1995). One effect has been to 'professionalise' what were previously volunteer roles by the employment of people who understand legal and financial issues. The transaction costs of prolonged contract negotiations are disproportionately large, and funding is highly volatile. Nine years later, Chouhan and Lusane (2004) examined how black and minority ethnic organisations worked with potential funders. They found that small organisations were hampered by stereotyping and unrealistic demands on administrative capacity. In particular, statutory agencies did not recognise the potential for social inclusion offered by support to developing community groups. The *Think Smart ... Think Voluntary Sector* initiative (OCG/Home Office, 2004) acknowledges a further ideological shift, with the voluntary and community sector now being seen in a compact as partners rather than simply as agents, with 'value for money' and innovation particularly highlighted as strengths. The report calls for a 'fundamental change of attitude' and the involvement of the voluntary sector not just in procurement, but in the shaping of services and the definition of outcomes.

Planning mechanisms

If government was seeking a cheaper option, community care never promised that it would cost less money overall than expanding residential care. The Audit Commission (1986, para. 13) made it quite clear from the outset that the total (although not the unit) cost of community care would be 'comparable with the cost of institutional care'. Government control over policy was, however, developed through the funding system, with transitional grant aid often linked to meeting performance targets, cooperating with other agencies and developing the workforce. The requirement to produce community care plans came to an end in 2003. Perhaps as a reflection of the greater strategic importance of healthcare services in delivering community care agendas, the main planning vehicle is now the health improvement and modernisation plan (HiMP) and the joint investment plan (JIP) to be produced by health and social care communities on a locality basis. Local strategic partnerships, often involving housing and leisure services as well as a range of independent sector providers, are also an important planning forum. However, social services authorities are still required to state their eligibility criteria and plans for adult care services in *Better Care, Higher Standards Guidance* charters (DoH, 1999c). Such charters will also include contact details of local voluntary organisations that provide support to users and carers.

Community care services

Section 47, the assessment section of the NHSCCA 1990, refers to an assessment for 'community care services'. The term 'community care services' is in itself a term of art with a literal legal meaning (McDonald, 2004). It does not mean any services that may be available to a person living in the community; strictly speaking, it means only those services which are defined as community care services in s.46(3) of the Act. This means services provided under:

- Part III of the National Assistance Act 1948
- Section 45 of the Health Services and Public Health Act 1968
- Section 21 of and Schedule 8 to the National Health Service Act 1977
- Section 117 of the Mental Health Act 1983.

Part III of the National Assistance Act 1948 refers in s.21 to the duty to provide residential accommodation for those 'in need of care and attention not otherwise available to them' and in s.29 to the power to provide services for people who are substantially and permanently disabled. Section 45 of the Health Services and Public Health Act 1968 gives a power (but not a duty) to local authorities to provide support for older people. The National Health Service Act 1977 again empowers a local authority to provide services to those suffering from or recovering from any type of illness, and also a duty to provide a home help service for their area. Section 117 of the Mental Health Act 1983 imposes aftercare duties in respect of people detained under section 3 of that Act, and some other sections. The important point to note is that the NHSCCA 1990 imposes no new substantive duties on local authorities to provide services that they were not already providing under existing legislation. There is some scope for innovation; for example drug and alcohol services and services to people with HIV/AIDS may be provided under section 21 and Schedule 8 of the National Health Service Act 1977. However, any expectation that the NHSCCA 1990 would of itself give an entitlement to a whole new range of services has proved to be illusory. The complexity of the current law and the failure in 1990 to review and modernise the relevant legislation is criticised by Clements (1996). Entitlement to service remains clouded by the distinction between powers and duties. The local authority has a duty to provide some services (such as residential care), while other services are discretionary, insofar as the local authority has only a power to provide them (meals on wheels, for example, or daycare for older people).

Assessment and provision of services

The appearance of need under section 47(1)(a) of the NHSCCA 1990 triggers the duty to assess – not any request for assessment as such. Section 47(1)(b) goes on to say that the local authority, having regard to the results of that assessment, shall then decide whether those needs call for the provision by them of any such service. As subsections (a) and (b) are conceptually distinct, it is clear that the process is a two-stage one: first, the assessment of presenting need and, second, a decision on the provision of services to meet eligible needs. Needs-led assessment, however, is not the same as user-led assessment; in other words, what people say they want or would like may not be the service that the local authority will provide. The *Managers' Guide* (SSI/DoH, 1991a, paras 12 and 13) emphasises the relativity of need:

Need is a dynamic concept, the definition of which will vary over time in accordance with:

■ changes in national legislation
■ changes in local policy
■ the availability of resources
■ the patterns of local demand.

The application of this definition in effect means that need may be defined as non-existent in circumstances where there are no resources to meet that need. So local authorities may restrict resources to people who present the greatest risks, who the most vulnerable or the least well supported by informal carers. The legality of this sort of policy was challenged in *R. v. Gloucestershire County Council, ex parte Barry* [1997] 2 WLR 459 (McDonald, 2004). The political background to this case was the decision by Gloucestershire County Council to withdraw (by letter) domestic cleaning and laundry facilities from 1,500 disabled people in its area. Although the withdrawal of services across the board without a formal reassessment in individual cases was held to be unlawful, the principle that services could be redistributed according to changing eligibility criteria was upheld. This is not to deny the necessity for assessment per se; it is clear that there are a number of factors as well as resources to be taken into account by the local authority in reaching its decision:

■ the nature and extent of the person's disability
■ the manner in which and the extent to which his quality of life would be improved by the service
■ the cost of the service, taking into account any financial assessment.

The local authority must also carry out its functions in a responsible manner; it cannot set eligibility criteria so unreasonably high that obviously needy people would be left without a service. Concern, however, that eligibility for services varied so widely across different parts of the country and could be inequitable between different user groups led to the publication in 2002 of *Fair Access to Care Services* (FACS) (DoH, 2002g), as guidance for local authorities to follow in deciding whether and how to meet assessed social care needs. FACS, as a manifestation of targeting especially vulnerable individuals whilst structuring local discretion, is discussed in Chapter 3.

Health service changes

The NHS has undergone profound changes over the past two decades which parallel those within social care. Change began in the mid-1980s with what was called 'the move to general management'. This sought to replace executive control of the NHS by clinicians with administration by professional managers, appointed for their management skills rather than their knowledge of patient care. But the basic principles of the NHS from its inception in 1948 remained intact; health services were to continue to be funded out of general taxation (as opposed to, say, an insurance system) and services would remain, on the whole, free at the point of delivery. The major divide within the system was between hospital services and community services; the latter provided by pharmacists, community nurses and GPs. The idea of a purchaser/provider split in healthcare stemmed from the White Paper *Working for Patients* (DoH, 1989). Although contemporaneous with the White Paper on community care (DoH, 1989b), relationships between the two systems, particularly in relation to the nursing needs of older people, those with disabilities and those with mental health problems living in the community, were not defined (Means and Smith, 1994). As SSDs became the lead authority for social care, the particular contribution of healthcare services to community care was not explored. This history of separate development has meant that the whole of the subsequent history of healthcare and social care has necessarily been one of the need for collaboration and consultation.

The NHSCCA 1990 did however bring in two major changes in respect of healthcare: the creation of NHS trusts and the opportunity for fundholding GP practices. Although the public nature of the NHS remained, an internal market was thereby created, within which NHS hospital and community trusts would provide services to be commissioned by health authorities undertaking a strategic planning role for their region. Services for individual patients would then be bought by GPs who, if they were fundholders, could choose their own providers, rather than having them chosen by the health authority. Contracts within the internal market were subject to a legal regime which was entirely their own. There is no real evidence that they increased patient power (Harden, 1992), and the internal market within the NHS has now been dismantled. *Shifting the Balance of Power within the NHS: Securing Delivery* (DoH, 2001) explains how primary care trusts (PCTs), as formal groupings of GPs and other community health services, were to become the lead organisation in assessing, planning and securing the range of healthcare services. Following negotiations between the NHS Confederation and the British Medical Association (BMA), a new contract for the provision of general medical services by GPs has been drawn up (www.nhsemployers.org). The contract, which GPs will enter into with PCTs locally, defines what are 'essential' and what are 'additional' and 'enhanced' services. It also enables GPs to opt out of out of hours services for the first time. The status of GPs as independent contractors within the NHS is maintained. As well as more complex clinical procedures, 'enhanced' services can include care for homeless people, services for patients who are alcohol or drug misusers and specialised care of patients with depression. The purchaser/provider split remains, to the extent that secondary and tertiary NHS services will still be commissioned through NHS trusts. The whole system is administered by strategic health authorities under the guidance of four new regional directors of health and social care. In furtherance of a patient-centred agenda, support for patients in dispute with healthcare providers is provided by the Patient Advice and Liaison Service (PALS) and patient forums are also represented on trust boards. The transformation of the NHS is discussed in greater detail in Chapter 10.

Education changes

Since the 1980s the provision of state-funded education has also been subject to the purchaser/provider split. The Education Act 1988 introduced local management of schools (LMS) and enabled individual schools to apply for grant-maintained status in order to control their own budgets independently of the LEA. Schools were also enabled to compete with each other to attract pupils and their success in public examinations was published in the form of league tables. Parents (if not pupils) have become consumers who can make choices between available schools.

Current government policy on education focuses on social inclusion, and thus impacts on social work practice at the interface of the two systems (Blyth, 2001). Low educational attainment by young people in care, the needs of young carers and school exclusion were topics of concern in the 1990s, within the context of greater competition between schools. At the same time, there was increasing evidence of the role of schools in the 'welfare network' and the positive contribution they could make to children, young people and families experiencing adversity. Key policies that have been retained and extended (Blyth, 2001) include:

- the use of market mechanisms as the bases of funding schools
- the managerialisation of education via the national curriculum and OFSTED inspection
- the encouragement of pedagogic traditionalism through testing and the literacy and numeracy strategies
- the promotion of parental responsibility for school attendance
- selective targeting of resources.

The 'new' aspects are an emphasis on achievement, social inclusion and integrated service provision. Examples of such services are Sure Start, as a support programme for the families of young children in disadvantaged areas, the development of youth offending teams, the Connexions service for 13–19-year-olds, education action zones and 'extended schools', offering social care as well as educational facilities. Changes to the Education Act 2002 have enabled extended schools directly to provide childcare, family learning, health and social care, lifelong learning opportunities, study support, sports and arts facilities (Sale, 2003). The promotion of schools as a community resource will enable social workers to do outreach work in schools, perhaps with children in the care system or those with special educational needs. It is also seen as enhancing professional relationships and enabling information to be shared (Winchester, 2001).

Ironically, the purchaser/provider split in education has produced particular difficulties in relation to pupils who have been 'statemented', where the LEA will have to contract both to meet the need for special educational provision and support services specified in the statement. Disputes between the LEA and parents are no longer a matter for internal resolution; appeal can be made to the Special Educational Needs and Disability Tribunal against a refusal to make a statement, as well as to challenge the content of the statement itself. This again is an instance of increasing legalism within administrative systems, which is paralleled by the use of legal sanctions against parents whose children truant from school, are excluded or display antisocial behaviour (McDonald, 2004).

Greater autonomy for high performing schools is a likely future development. It will be made easier for schools to borrow money or enter into partnerships with business. City academies will be independent of LEA control, operating effectively as state-funded independent schools. The future for education therefore appears to be more pluralism, more choice for parents and an entrepreneurial approach to development. Education, however, is not confined to schooling. The *Practitioners' Guide* (SSI/DoH, 1991) makes it clear that assessment of educational needs, broadly defined, is an essential element of a comprehensive assessment. Social workers as assessors have an obligation to be proactive in referring on to appropriate agencies for educational needs to be met but social work agencies also have a legal duty to provide supportive care services. Also, in line with the greater emphasis on equal opportunities to combat social exclusion, the receipt of welfare benefits (see Chapter 9) may be dependent upon undergoing training as part of the New Deal in employment.

Housing

Good quality housing is a necessary but not sufficient condition for effective community care. Many people would choose to remain in their own homes, if necessary adaptations could be made for acquired disabilities, and the idea of 'lifetime homes' and assistive technology has become an important issue in building design. Movement out of institutions also depends on suitable accommodation being available; but suitable in this context will include the availability of good support services as well as bricks and mortar. The contribution of housing to community care is further discussed in Chapter 11.

In social policy terms, the movement has been away from direct local authority provision of housing stock towards the development of housing associations as providers of care. Public subsidy has come to be provided in the form of means-tested housing benefit. Although the Housing Act 1996 addressed the problem of homelessness by placing more emphasis on personal responsibility, the Homelessness Act 2002 has put into place the partnership agenda by requiring authorities to work together in the production and implementation of homelessness plans. Advocating on behalf of homeless and vulnerable people will become a more complex task for social workers, as they strike a balance between stressing the need for accommodation without overemphasising potential problems that the resident may pose in housing management terms. For their part, housing authorities will legitimately be looking to community care assessments for care services to complement support services to vulnerable residents, more recently formalised under the *Supporting People* (ODPM, 2003) initiative.

Social services authorities are themselves sources of accommodation under Part III National Assistance Act 1948. Section 21 of that Act imposes a duty to provide residential accommodation 'to persons in need of care and attention not otherwise available to them'. There has recently been an upsurge of interest in the reinterpretation of the National Assistance Act 1948 as a potential source of support for asylum seekers who are otherwise excluded from the public housing sector and the social security benefits system. This has led Clements (1996) to see SSDs as performing the function of a residual welfare net to fill the gaps left by other agencies or government policy.

The social security system

The Department of Social Security has had its functions transferred to the appropriately named Department for Work and Pensions (DWP). What was perceived as passive dependency on welfare benefits has recently been supplemented by the introduction of tax credits as an incentive to move from welfare into work and to reward medium-range earners and savers. Although the benefits system is administered according to national rules laid down in legislation and guidance, some parts of the system, for example the social fund (see Chapter 9), contain a significant element of local discretion. There is little coordination between the benefits system and community care systems, even though many recipients of community care services have social security benefits as their sole source of income, and some benefits, such as disability living allowance, are based on social as well as medical need. The introduction of charges for domiciliary care and direct payments accelerated the process of seeing care as a commodity to be bought and sold. Although social workers have acknowledged the importance of welfare rights advice to maximise income, they have generally shown a reluctance to become enmeshed in financial issues. Yet financial issues raise fundamental questions around the basic values of confidentiality, family responsibility and personal autonomy, which raise real dilemmas for social workers (Bradley and Manthorpe, 1995). Some of these dilemmas will be further addressed in Chapter 9.

The criminal justice system

Since the Criminal Justice Act 1991, the emphasis within the criminal justice system has been increasingly offence-based. There is less emphasis on the personal characteristics of the offender or welfare issues. Community care assessments are of relevance, however, at a number of points in the process. In some parts of the country, diversionary schemes exist to interview people arrested by the police who may appear to be dealt with more appropriately by social services authorities. Social workers or community mental health nurses may also attend magistrates' courts to identify individuals going through the criminal justice process. The identification of drug and alcohol problems associated with offending behaviour has become an important part of the work of the Probation Service as part of the National Offender Management Service which may work with voluntary agencies in providing individual or groupwork programmes. Prisoners anticipating release are also entitled to an appropriate assessment if they appear to be in need of community care services. This is an important link because the outcome of a parole hearing may depend on support being available in the community, and prisoners released on licence may need housing, welfare rights advice and in some cases specialist services from community teams.

Youth offending teams have become a model for interdisciplinary working by their employment of social workers, police, healthcare professionals and educationalists, amongst others, to deliver integrated services to young people. Increasingly, their work is of a preventive but authoritarian nature and involves linking young people with community support services. The meeting of targets is enforced through national standards, whilst assessments and the delivery of direct interventions with individuals or groups follow pro forma checklists and scripted care plans. There are parallels here with contemporaneous changes in the delivery of services to adults under community care towards greater managerial control through the specification of tasks and outcomes.

The challenge for social work

Sheppard (1995, p. vii) regards community care as 'the greatest challenge to social work for at least 20 years'. He identifies elements of both continuity and change. The change is in the threat to professionalism with the bureaucratisation of social care and the inclusion of market principles. The continuity lies in the relevance of core social work approaches: interpersonal skills; working with social networks and social supports; and task-centred practice. What is likely to be diminished is 'sentimental work' such as counselling, in which the client sets the agenda, and the traditional casework approach, in which the relationship is seen as the major factor in therapeutic work (Strauss, 1964).

The focused nature of care management is however a development to be welcomed. As long ago as 1979, Goldberg and Warburton were critical of long-term and often aimless casework and surveillance, especially with children and families but also with physically disabled and older people. Intermittent long-term support, punctuated by hectic activity in times of crisis, rarely results in any change of behaviour for personal growth. If the focus is to be on personal change, a sustained but time-limited relationship within which clients feel safe enough to confront emotional problems can lead to a less crisis-ridden existence and in some cases to behavioural changes (Mattison and Sinclair, 1979). Similarly, Goldberg and Warburton (1979) found that monitoring and review visiting was the predominant social work activity with older people allocated to long-term teams. Yet in over two-thirds of the cases surveyed, unanticipated illness or frailty occurred before the next planned review. In these circumstances, maintaining contact through provider services, developing community networks for support or early warning of deterioration would be more effective than periodic but sustained social worker visits. By enabling such networks to develop and focusing the involvement of care management on strategic issues, community care policies are less likely to allow such drift to happen.

How do social workers experience practice in community care?

What has been the impact of policy changes on practice? Has worker satisfaction declined as discretion arguably has been reduced? Fook (2002) identifies a managerialist discourse which has ousted the professional discourse, formerly identified with casework. This in turn has had an impact on case (or care) management as a system, since:

> in a climate of increased government and management control over professionals and service users, it is likely that case management is a practice which will:
>
> ■ be system rather than service user focused
> ■ serve management rather than professional or service user interests
> ■ be technocratic and simplistic rather than complex, holistic or long term
> ■ be driven by an economic, rationalist imperative. (Fook, 2002, p. 149)

The NISW research programme 1992–97 found that for all staff working in social care, satisfaction was gained from services delivered, but was marred by both structural and personal factors: workplace stress; abuse and violence from service users and their relatives; racism from service users and colleagues; and changes in the workplace (Balloch and McLean, 2000). There are well evidenced links between personal and professional satisfaction and agency efficiency. The Social Services Inspectorate (SSI, 2003) identified the most effective services as those where frontline social workers are supported in a clear managerial framework and where they are encouraged to develop reflective practice and improve their professional skills in making judgements in complex situations, quoting the *Victoria Climbié Inquiry* report's finding (Laming, 2003, p. 357) that practice should be governed by professional judgement, not by rules and procedures. Typically, councils performing poorly in social care:

■ show limited political commitment to social services, avoid difficult decisions, and do not determine or resource strategic priorities
■ do not consult service users and carers effectively
■ fail to support staff, develop an effective workforce strategy, or operate an effective quality assurance system
■ fail to agree a joint strategy with partners – especially health partners.

Conversely, high performers are characterised by a tendency to 'locate their social care performance in the context of a vision of local well-being' (SSI, 2003, para. 2.10). This accords with Jordan's (2000) vision of a new conception of public social services more firmly rooted in neighbourhoods and linked with community groups, and less concerned with enforcement and surveillance – but only if communities are seen as a source of economic and social regeneration, and not as a system of social control.

The 'success' of the purchaser/provider split, however, has had the effect of moving professional involvement away from direct face-to-face work and into specialised roles around the assessment of resources and risks, the investigation of abuse and rule-breaking and the setting up and enforcement of contracts (Jordan, 2000, p. 37). More commercial organisations, employing fewer trained social workers, have moved into service provision. Voluntary and private sector providers now employ two-thirds of social care staff (Balloch and McLean, 2000);

between 1997 and 2002, the number of whole-time equivalent staff employed directly by SSDs fell by 9 per cent (SSI, 2003). A change in philosophy under New Labour, however, has meant that less reliance is placed on the ability of market forces per se to effect change, and more emphasis is placed on the raising of standards by government authorisation of independent sector services and duties of cooperation with other statutory sector services such as health and housing (Malin et al., 2002).

Organisational responsibility for standards of professional practice has been introduced with the creation of the General Social Care Council (GSCC), with its registration powers and codes of practice not only for individual workers, but also for employers engaged as learning organisations. Similarly, within the NHS, organisational responsibility for standards of professional practice is included within the system of clinical governance, as an *Organisation with a Memory* (DoH, 2000). Parton et al.'s (1997) view of risk as governing the relationship between the responsibilities of state agents and private individuals has increasingly come to govern both day-to-day practice and decision-making, particularly through the modification of systems and procedures for identifying risk factors and managing the risks thus identified. Kemshall (2002, p. 88) sees this as introducing a 'prudentialism' into social work practice, whereby 'eligibility for provision is no longer needs-led and preventative, it is entirely investigative, forensic and risk-based'. *Fair Access to Care Services* (DoH, 2002g), with its emphasis on the banding of eligibility criteria according to risk, feeds into this organisational structuring of social work discretion, arguably as another mechanism for 'risk insurance' (Parton et al., 1997). This greater government and management control over professional practice will, according to Fook (2002, p. 149), ignore the real complexities of decision-making in favour of:

> increased possibilities that individual professional workers or case managers, whatever their occupational background, will take the brunt of the blame/responsibility for the effectiveness of the case management process; regardless of the level and appropriateness of the resourcing available or authority they hold.

The ramifications of this statement for social work practice will be explored in subsequent chapters, as the National Occupational Standards for social work are described in relation to the process of care management.

Concluding comments

The new philosophy and language of community care has spread beyond the provision of social care services to inform the work of a range of statutory agencies. Economic policy and managerial rather than professional orientations continue to inform service delivery. This has inevitably had an impact on the experience of individual workers and service users and evidence from research and inspections of care services needs to be examined to see how social work practice has changed as community care has developed.

PAUSE AND REFLECT

Choose one of these areas of policy:

Education
Housing
Social security
Criminal justice

Consider the points of contact between these services and community care services that are necessary in order to support individuals or communities in an integrated way. You could consider, for example, the needs of children with disabilities for education and support, the housing needs of ex-prisoners or assistance to people with mental health problems to sustain employment. From your own experience, how might services be improved in your area of choice?

CASE STUDY

Opportunities and barriers
John Finch is 16 years old, has Down syndrome and has always received special schooling. He lives with his mother Katie, who is a single parent and does not work. John leaves school in two years' time.

What formal systems need to work together in order to ensure a good transition into adulthood for John? What barriers may exist to John and his mother receiving the sort of service and opportunities that they may feel they need?

FURTHER READING

Hudson, B. (ed.) *The Changing Role of Social Care* (2000). London: Jessica Kingsley.
Updates the development of social care policy to *Modernising Social Services* and also looks at variations across the UK. Contains chapters on social care, housing and social security.

Lewis, J. and Glennerster, H. (1996) *Implementing the New Community Care*. Buckingham: Open University Press.
Looks at the differential application of community care policy in different local authorities from the perspective of practitioners and managers.

CHAPTER 3

Needs-led Assessment

Introduction

Good quality assessment is the cornerstone of effective social work practice, whatever the setting. For social workers, the major impact of the NHSCCA 1990 is to place assessment for community care services on a statutory basis, so that what social workers may legitimately claim to be doing when they are carrying out an assessment is statutory work; work which demands the highest priority and the greatest degree of expertise. One consequence of doing statutory work is that it is the legal interpretation of the assessment process which is all-important; it is more compelling than departmental policy and procedures, which are at best interpretations of legal powers and duties (McDonald, 1997).

This chapter considers the statutory framework within which assessment takes place and examines the dilemmas inherent in assessing need within the context of increasingly scarce resources. The reader is reminded that community care assessment may become relevant in contexts other than adult care, for example within work with children and families where there are mental health problems or disability issues, or in a criminal justice context. A community care assessment in these circumstances can act as a gateway to a wide range of other services. The generic nature of assessment work is therefore emphasised. Skills needed in assessment are explained, both according to a due process model and for the development of partnership in practice between the agency and the service user. Assessment of carers' needs is also included here. The fundamental question throughout is: what is a need and who legitimately defines it as such? Examining the statutory framework is a good place to begin to try to answer this question, and to explain the scope of National Occupational Standards key role 1.

KEY ROLE I

Prepare for and work with individuals, families, carers, groups and communities to assess their needs and circumstances

The statutory framework

Section 47(1) of the NHSCCA 1990 emphasises that assessment is a 'service' in its own right that the local authority is under a duty to provide, irrespective of whether services are available or indeed asked for. It is also clear that the local authority should take the initiative in providing assessments. The duty to assess is not dependent on a request being made, but on the local authority deciding that it appears to it that a person may be in need of services. This is important at the initial screening or referral stage where an individual will often phrase his request in terms of an ineligible service, for example help with domestic cleaning. This does not disentitle that person to an assessment of his need for other services (which further investigation may reveal). Disseminating information, the first task within care management, thus shades into assessment at this point.

What is assessment?

Veronica Coulshed (1991, p. 30) gives a succinct definition of assessment: 'an assessment is a perceptual/analytical process of selecting, categorising, organising and synthesising data'. In other words, assessment is an intellectual process which seeks to make sense of the world by gathering together, interpreting and processing information relevant to the issue or problem under scrutiny.

The emphasis on assessment as ongoing stresses the dynamic nature of the process; as new information is gathered, or situations change, so the assessment will change. An assessment therefore is basically a working hypothesis for action. It is not a process which is confined to individuals. Specht and Vickery (1977) introduce the idea of a unified assessment which may be applied to individuals, groups, neighbourhoods, organisations and the wider environment. This sort of approach is particularly suited to a care management model of social work, as it seeks to address, in the round, the answers to the following questions:

- what is the problem?
- who is the client?
- what are the goals?
- who or what has to be changed or influenced, in order to meet the goals?
- what are the tasks and roles of the social worker?

Of course, the answers to these questions can never be objectively determined. They all to a greater or lesser extent depend on: the theoretical orientation of workers; their professional perspective; their degree of knowledge about this and comparable situations; their value system; and the synthesis of the relationship between worker and client. Macdonald (1991) stresses the importance in assessment of emphasising strengths, rather than problems. To begin with a deficit model may act as a powerful negative interpreter of all subsequent actions in the light of that model.

The assessment process

Source materials for putting together an assessment may be diverse. They may come from agency files, other professionals, interviews with clients and interviews with carers. The *Managers' Guide* (SSI/DoH, 1991a, p. 46) is explicit about the administrative knowledge base required. In order to undertake an assessment of need, staff have to know:

- the needs for which the agency accepts responsibility
- the needs for which other care agencies accept responsibility
- the needs of carers which qualify for assistance
- the agency's priorities in responding to need
- the financial assessment criteria for determining user's contributions
- the agency's policy on risk to the user and to the community
- the legal requirements.

This emphasis in assessment on the dichotomies between need/risk, strengths/ resources and users/carers is something taken up by Hughes (1993), and she describes a framework for the assessment of older people which utilises these categories to map out the different elements of a situation and the perspectives of the participants within it. Particular domains of assessment may now be highlighted in the NSFs for older people and mental health. The particular knowledge that the social worker will bring to the situation is not simply knowledge of legislation and guidance, but knowledge of sources of risk and harm, whether individual or structural, knowledge of systems and knowledge of the impact of change, loss or gain on people and relationships (Coulshed and Orme, 1998).

Emphasis is on needs-led rather than resource-led assessment, that is, on an assessment which is based on individual interpretations of need rather than the matching of people to resources. This is not, however, the same as user-led assessment, where the individual defines his or her own care needs without professional interpretation. The *Practitioners' Guide* (SSI/DoH, 1991, para. 3.35) makes it clear that assessment in community care must be professionally determined: 'Ultimately, however, having weighed the views of all parties, including his/her own observation, the assessing practitioner is responsible for defining the user's needs.' A due process model is acknowledged, however, as practitioners must ensure that users understand:

- what is involved in the assessment procedures
- the likely timescale
- what authority the practitioner holds
- their entitlement to information, participation and representation. (SSI/DoH, 1991a, para. 3.16)

It is therefore the responsibility of the worker to guide people through the assessment process. This requires a range of interpersonal skills to encourage people to explore often difficult areas of their lives and relationships under circumstances of stress. There is a wide literature available on the identification and use of interpersonal skills, for example Rogers (1967); Burnard (1989); Egan (1990); Trevithick (2000).

Skills in assessment

A study of users' perceptions of helping skills (Harding and Beresford, 1996) emphasised the importance of the following skills:

- listening and communicating
- counselling and understanding
- knowledge about local services
- enabling and negotiating
- a sense of judgement about risks.

All these are basic and enduring social work skills. Particular skills may be needed in interviewing people with different needs, for example people whose language of choice is not English or those with sensory impairments. Workers will need to be aware of their own value base and assumptions, which may not reflect the experiences of people who live with poverty or racism as part of their daily lives (Cameron et al., 1996). In interviewing older people, the complex relationship between age, poverty and the use of language – 'I'm just managing' – is explored by Barrett (1996). How language is used as a coping or defence mechanism needs to be understood not only in a historical context of avoiding 'the welfare' or 'the workhouse', but for its continuing relevance to the marginalisation of older people through poverty and ageism when scarce resources are to be allocated (Robertson, 1995).

The interaction between assessors and service users is seen by Smale and Tuson (1993) as fitting one of three models:

1. The *questioning model* – the assessor sets the agenda and is perceived as the 'expert'
2. The *administrative model* – pro formas are drawn up by managers to constrain both users and professionals
3. The *exchange model* – the assessment process is embarked on as a shared enterprise, and the user is respected as the expert on himself or herself.

The exchange model, where both parties together construct their own agenda, is clearly the means by which stereotypical assumptions may be avoided and strengths as well as deficits acknowledged.

Assessment and working in partnership

Smale and Tuson's (1993) exchange model of assessment fits well with Marsh and Fisher's (1992) agenda for developing partnership in practice between the agency and the client. Marsh and Fisher's principles of partnership are that:

- Investigations of problems must be with the explicit consent of the potential user(s) and client(s). Where there is no consent, investigations should be kept to the minimum, consistent with statutory responsibilities.
- User agreement or a clear statutory mandate are the only bases of partnership-based intervention.

- Intervention must be based on the values of all relevant family members and carers.
- Services must be based on negotiated agreement, rather than assumptions or prejudices concerning the behaviour and wishes of users.
- Users must have the greatest possible degree of choice in the services they are offered.

Working in partnership thus demands openness and honesty about the purpose of the intervention and its legal basis. The scope of the assessment will, however, be a matter for negotiation. The approach is respectful of persons, insofar as it protects them from intrusive questioning about personal issues which are not strictly necessary for the fulfilment of the legal mandate. The emphasis on negotiated agreement seeks to avoid, or at least clarify, assumptions that may be brought to the assessment concerning, for example, the obligations of carers, the culture of the family or the allocation of gender roles. Agreement need not necessarily be explicit; it can be inferred from behaviour, for example in a positive response given by a person with dementia to a first introduction to a day centre. The last requirement, that potential users should have the greatest possible degree of choice, is allied to openness about why particular services might not be available. Giving people a written care plan which includes unmet need is part of this process of enabling people to measure what they believe to have been agreed against the actual service provided.

Determining the level of assessment

Determining the level of assessment, that is, differentiating between straightforward requests for services and requests which need more complex assessment, is seen as a management task and is the second stage of the care management process. The *Managers' Guide* (SSI/DoH, 1991a) differentiates between six different levels of assessment, ranging from simple (single service) to comprehensive. Specialist assessments may be provided by other people within or outside the social work team, such as occupational therapists. Comprehensive assessments cover all potential areas of need and are multidisciplinary in nature.

The *Community Care Assessment Directions* (DoH, 2004) place existing good practice and guidance on conducting care assessments and care planning into a legal framework by requiring full involvement of individuals and their carers. The directions also state that assessments for all adults with complex needs should take account of physical, cognitive, behavioural and social participation needs. Assessment of healthcare and housing needs (so far as they are relevant) will necessitate referral on to the appropriate healthcare body or housing authority, inviting them to assist 'to such extent as is reasonable in the circumstances, in the making of the assessment' (s.47(3) NHSCCA 1990). This is obviously an important provision for determining the viability of interprofessional assessments, when the complementary provision of services is often crucial in putting together a package of care. Attempts to compel cooperation by legal action have proved unsuccessful. As each authority is charged by statute with its own sphere of action, so they are competent to set their own internal priorities for service. This has been seen most clearly in disputes between SSDs and housing departments in respect of provision for homeless families and asylum seekers (Clements, 2004).

Service users who are disabled will find it advantageous to stress the disability aspect of their situation when approaching assessment. If, at any time during the assessment under s.47(1) of the 1990 Act, it appears to the local authority that the person being assessed is a disabled person, s.47(2) requires the local authority to make a decision as to the services he/she requires as mentioned in section 4 of the Disabled Persons (Services, Consultation and Representation) Act 1986. This seems a complicated provision; bringing in a different assessment regime for people who are disabled which diverges from the mainstream assessment under section 47. Why should it be beneficial for people to be dealt with under the Disabled Persons Act 1986? The answer is that the Disabled Persons Act 1986 is the way into a list of services for disabled people, including the provision of aids and adaptations, daycare, domiciliary care and holiday provision, which is set out in section 2 of the Chronically Sick and Disabled Persons Act 1970. The 1970 Act, which in its day pioneered the idea of rights for disabled people, has been criticised for its 'service list' approach to services compared to the needs-led approach of the 1990 Act. However, as the needs-led approach has become constrained by resource limitations and strict eligibility criteria, the rights-based approach of the 1970 Act has again been in the ascendant because of the specificity of services contained within it and the availability of a personal right of action for its breach (McDonald, 1997).

Fair Access to Care Services

Fair Access to Care Services: Guidance on Eligibility Criteria for Adult Social Care (DoH, 2002g) is part of the centralisation of control over local authority discretion. The FACS guidance is intended to lead to fairer and more consistent eligibility criteria across the country. Using a framework based on cumulative functional capacity, there are four eligibility bands:

- *Critical*   – when life or vital social roles are threatened, significant health problems have developed or where there is serious abuse or neglect.
- *Substantial* – when choice or control over the immediate environment is substantially limited, for example by an inability to carry out the majority of personal care tasks or domestic routines.
- *Moderate* – when there is, or will be, an inability to carry out several personal care tasks or domestic routines.
- *Low*   – when there is, or will be, in inability to carry out one or two personal care tasks or domestic routines.

The bands will apply to eligibility for community care services following assessment under s.47 NHSCCA 1990. The threshold for assessment for what are called 'presenting' needs (as opposed to 'eligible' needs) for services remains low. The guidance makes it clear that local authorities should not operate eligibility criteria for the type and depth of assessment that they carry out and should not screen individuals out of the assessment process before sufficient information is known about them. The core principle is that councils should operate just one eligibility decision for all adults seeking social care support: that is, should people be helped or not? They should not operate eligibility criteria for specific services such as home care or daycare. Implementation of the guidance will help to ensure that where it has been decided to provide services, people with similar assessed needs should receive services that deliver equivalent *outcomes,* no matter where they live or what user group they may be identified as belonging to. So, discrimination on the grounds of age, race, gender or disability should be addressed in the implementation of the guidance. Prevention and longer term needs as well as immediate requirements should also be addressed in the drawing up of eligibility criteria. As the guidance focuses on 'roles' as well as 'tasks', individuals with parenting responsibilities should be able to access services under FACS, as well as being eligible for assessment under the *Framework for the Assessment of Children in Need and their Families* (DoH, 2000a).

What are needs?

Doyal and Gough (1990) point to the absence of a clear and detailed theory of human need on which accurate need assessment can be based. There is no metalegal right of citizenship which contains within it a catalogue of those needs which must be satisfied in order to enable optimal social participation; indeed, shifting political and economic circumstances make a consensus on need controversial. Assessment systems are about procedural models of need – how to get what is available. In this context, Braye and Preston-Shoot (1995) see needs, rights and resources as a triangulation, the invocation of any one of which can be countered by the tensions arising between the other two.

The *Practitioners' Guide* (SSI/DoH, 1991, para. 11) defines needs as the shorthand for:

> the requirements of individuals to enable them to achieve, maintain or restore an acceptable level of social independence or quality of life, as defined by the particular care agency or authority.

Need is thus seen as a relative concept. In the context of community care, need has to be defined at the local level. That definition sets limits to the discretion of practitioners in accessing resources (SSI/DoH, 1991, para. 13). In other words, the assessment process is seen to reflect Smale and Tuson's managerial typology, within which conformity to preset eligibility criteria triggers 'need' and professional discretion is at a minimum.

A resource-led definition of need at the assessment stage compromises professionalism; is the occupational therapist constrained never to assess a need for a bathroom adaptation, because all that is available is bath boards and bath seats? If so, there would be no concept of unmet need for local authorities to be cautious of recording. The Laming letter advised local authorities to aggregate unmet 'preferences' rather than unmet need in such a way that individuals could not be identified, so as to avoid legal challenges. Such an approach is unacceptable to service users. Responding to the NISW survey *The Standards We Expect* (Harding and Beresford, 1996), the Wiltshire User Network stated: 'not recording unmet need is a disservice to us service users. Armed with information, we can have the evidence to complain.' Without some means of recording unmet need, the cyclical process within care management of using information on unmet need to inform service planning cannot be achieved. Certainly the practice guidance makes it clear that a care plan should contain details of 'any unmet needs with reasons – to be separately notified to the service planning system' (SSI/DoH, 1991, para. 4.32), although as Clements (2004) points out, FACS avoids any discussion of unmet need by distinguishing needs that are 'presented' by service users and needs that are 'eligible' for a service.

Recording and record-keeping

How, and by whom, contacts, assessments and care plans are recorded gives a powerful message about the partnership status accorded to professionals and service users. Signing and receiving a copy of the care plan enables services actually received to be checked against assessed needs and legal requirements. Recording should distinguish fact from opinion. For example, a comment that someone's house is unclean or that they are aggressive is simply an opinion. The actual state of the house or description of their behaviour, although it may be chosen selectively, is more readily accepted as an objective statement of fact. For people with a fragmented life history, agency records are an important storehouse of their past, and so great care should be taken that the material contained therein is accurate and contains positive as well as negative information.

Interprofessional working necessitates a new approach to assessment. Shared records may facilitate work by different professionals within the same agency. Different line management systems and different interpretations of statutory responsibility may mean that recording has to incorporate the referral of information between systems. Issues of confidentiality then come into play. Medical personnel in particular may be reluctant to pass on information without the consent of the patient, except where there is an obvious risk to the patient him/herself or some identifiable other person (BMA/Law Society, 2003). This approach is also apparent in the protection from disclosure without consent of third party information under the Data Protection Act 1998. Now all agency records should be written and organised with the possibility in mind of future access by the service user.

Freedom of information and data protection

Section 19 of the Freedom of Information Act 2000 requires public authorities to adopt and maintain a publication scheme which lists the information, for example policies and procedures, that the organisation has in its possession, together with the contact details of those people within the organisation who hold that information. The scheme was fully operational from 1 January 2005 and enables members of the public to know how public services, such as local authorities and the NHS, are organised and run, how much they cost and how complaints about services can be made.

The Freedom of Information Act does not, however, change the rights of service users to protection of their client confidentiality in accordance with Article 8 of the European Convention on Human Rights, the Data Protection Act 1998 and at common law. The Data Protection Act applies to paper records and computer-held data, and covers any information or 'personal data' that relates to an identifiable individual. There are eight principles of 'good information handling' with which data controllers must comply. These state that data must be:

- fairly and lawfully processed
- processed for limited purposes
- adequate, relevant and not excessive
- accurate
- not kept for longer than is necessary
- processed in conformity with the data subject's rights
- secure
- not transferred to countries outside the EU without adequate protection.

The Act makes a distinction between personal data and *sensitive* personal data such as racial or ethnic origin, religious beliefs, health and criminal convictions. Sensitive data can only be processed with the explicit consent of the data subject, if required by law, or to protect the vital interests of the data subject. A lack of clarity about the circumstances in which information can or should be shared between agencies is compounded by social workers not being clear with clients about why certain information is needed or what will be done with it (DoH, 2001d; Valois, 2002). Such a lack of clarity was an important factor in the Bichard Inquiry Report (2004) and in the Climbié inquiry in respect of child protection, with Lord Laming, the chair, making the following comment in his summary (Laming, 2003 p. 12):

> I was told that the free exchange of information about children and families about whom there are concerns is inhibited by the legislation on data protection and human rights. It appears that, unless a child is deemed to be in need of protection, information cannot be shared between agencies without staff running the risk of contravening this legislation. This has two consequences: either it deters information sharing, or it artificially increases concerns in order that they can be expressed as the need for protection. This is a matter that government must address. It is not a matter than can be tackled satisfactorily at local level.

In a different context, sharing information is fundamental to the introduction of the single assessment process with the NSF for older people (DoH, 2001a). Clearly, sharing information is critical for interagency work, but at the present time may well be hampered by a complex and unclear legal framework.

Assessment of carers

Providing proper support for carers was stated to be one of the cornerstones of community care policy, as outlined in the White Paper of 1989 (DoH, 1989a). Campaigning by the carers' movement has endeavoured to formalise this commitment. The 2001 census found that in England and Wales there were 5.2 million carers (approximately 10 per cent of the population). Caring was defined as:

> looking after or giving help or support to family members, friends, neighbours or others because of long term physical or mental ill health or disability, or problems related to old age.

Twenty one per cent of the total were heavy end carers, caring for 50 or more hours per week. Support for carers is a national priority and the National Carers Strategy (http://www.carers.gov.uk) identifies the following as rights for carers:

- the freedom to have a life of their own
- time for themselves
- the opportunity to continue work
- control over their life and the support they need
- better health and well-being
- integration into the community and peace of mind.

The Carers and Disabled Children Act 2000 has given carers, including carers of disabled children, who provide a substantial amount of care on a regular basis, a right to a free-standing assessment of their ability to provide or continue to provide care. Section 2 of the Act enables local authorities to provide carers services to those who are caring for adults. Such services may be provided by way of direct payments and there is also a power to issue vouchers for the purchase of respite provision. The term 'regular and substantial' is defined in guidance (DoH, 2001h) in relation to the impact of the caring role on the individual carer; this may include: length of time spent caring; age of the carer; demands of other roles as a parent or employee; and the sustainability of the carer role. There should be a focus on outcomes and a written care plan. Process issues identified include telling carers of their right to request an assessment, respecting confidentiality and separate recording of interviews where conflicts of interest arise.

The guidance does not explore the ramifications of Twigg's (1989) typology of how social workers view carers, which may highlight the ambivalences in their relationship; are they co-workers or a resource? Are they clients in their own right? The Carers (Equal Opportunities) Act 2004 stresses the independent status of carers by requiring their wish to be in employment and take part in leisure activities to be included in any assessment of need. The *Community Care Assessment Directions* (DoH, 2004d) also require local authorities to retain a written account of why it is felt inappropriate to involve the carer in an assessment of the person for whom they care. Separate guidance (DoH, 2002d) is more explicit; such carers are to be regarded as 'co-experts' and are entitled to an assessment of their caring needs, set out in a care plan.

Young carers

It has been estimated that there are approximately 50,000 young carers carrying out significant caring tasks and assuming a level of responsibility for another person which would usually be taken by an adult (Aldridge and Becker, 1993). The appropriate legislative framework for the provision of services to children is the Children Act 1989. However, the provision of community care services to adults should ensure that young carers are not expected to carry inappropriate levels of caring responsibilities. Social workers will need to take a family perspective when considering the needs of carers. A lack of generic training should not result in a narrow view of responsibility for either the child or the adult. Instead, the views of both should be considered, and there should be a readiness to refer adults to services appropriate to their needs. The contribution of mental health, disability or drug and alcohol services to the welfare of children in a household through the targeting of adults should not be underestimated. There may be situations in which individual casework or counselling is appropriate and those in which only structural or organisational change can offer any solution. For carers, this organisational view may lead to the development of carers groups or new services, such as night sitting. Working with carers challenges social workers to explore a range of methods of intervention which will include working with families as a group as well as looking at community support.

The overlap between adult and children's services in terms of need is substantial. Thoburn et al. (1995) found that 20 per cent of child protection cases in their research sample involved a parent or carer with a mental health problem. Problems of liaison, leading to a recommendation for specialist workers, were also researched by Stanley et al. (2003). Booth and Booth (1994), in their seminal study of parents with learning difficulties, emphasised the importance of community support in assisting parents to meet the developmental needs of the child. Guidance from the Advisory Council on the Misuse of Drugs (2003) links effective interventions for parental drug misuse to the welfare of the child. At an operational level, Horwath (2003) identifies the importance of organisational frameworks through the development of protocols and practice guidance in respect of both family support and child protection. Such liaison will be increasingly important as children's services diverge into children's trusts, local authorities appoint separate directors of children's services and services for children develop within a separate NSF.

Concluding comments

This chapter explored the meaning of assessment, using knowledge and skills in understanding individuals and their social situations. It also introduced the statutory framework within which decision-making will take place, and government guidance on the interpretation of need. Translating such understanding into plans for action is the focus of Chapter 4. A range of skills are required here, from business skills in accessing resources to skills in negotiation and recording. Professional dilemmas of empowerment versus protection and support versus care are explored. The chapter introduces key role 2, by focusing on the preparation, production and implementation of plans with individuals, families, carers, groups, communities and professional colleagues. It also explores units within key role 4 on the assessment and management of risk.

PAUSE AND REFLECT

1. Consider how you might use a 'carer's diary' as a way of enabling carers to contribute to their own assessment.
2. Consider how social workers in adult care might identify and respond to the needs of children within the family unit.

CASE STUDY

Assessment

Mrs Daisy Cotton is 75 years old and lives with her daughter Rose, aged 40, who has Down syndrome. They are not in receipt of any social care services from the statutory or independent sectors. Mrs Cotton has been informed that she needs to be admitted to hospital for a hysterectomy within the next four weeks. She says that she will not go unless proper arrangements can be made for Rose. Mrs Cotton's GP makes the referral, and the case is allocated to you as social worker.

How would you approach the assessment? With whom would you speak? What would be the short-term and long-term goals of assessment?

FURTHER READING

Crisp, B., Anderson, M., Orme, J. and Green Lister, P. (2003) *Learning and Teaching in Social Work Education: Knowledge Review I*. Bristol: SCIE/Policy Press.
The first of SCIE's Knowledge Reviews to support the new social work degree looks at assessment and the social work curriculum and gathers examples of best practice. There are extensive references and a literature review identifying papers which describe the teaching of assessment in social work and cognate disciplines.

Milner, J. and O'Byrne, P. (2002) *Assessment in Social Work* (2nd edn). Basingstoke: Palgrave Macmillan.
A classic text which analyses the task of assessment from different theoretical perspectives, for example psychoanalytic, task-centred, solution-focused. Written in an accessible style, highlighting the importance of social work values and anti-discriminatory practice in assessment.

Nolan, M. and Caldock, K. (1996) 'Assessment: identifying the barriers to good practice', *Health and Social Care in the Community*, **4**, pp 77–85.
Sets out a framework of good practice in assessment for adult care services using a person-centred model.

CHAPTER 4

Care Planning

Introduction

This chapter introduces the process of care planning and implementation. Formulating the care plan is the fourth stage of care management, the aim of which is: 'to identify the most appropriate ways of achieving the objectives identified by the assessment of need and incorporate them into an individual care plan' (SSI/DoH, 1991 p. 61). Issues of risk and protection, and support and care will be discussed as professional dilemmas within the agendas of care planning. Meeting needs and agreeing service objectives are discussed in the context of limited resources and a higher profile for financial considerations. This chapter focuses on the following key roles within National Occupational Standards.

KEY ROLE 2

Plan, carry out, review and evaluate social work practice with individuals, families, carers, groups, communities and other professionals

KEY ROLE 4

Manage risk to individuals, families, carers, groups, communities, self and colleagues

The care planning process

A care plan is a blueprint for action designed by the social worker and service user which follows on from assessment and which, according to the *Practitioners' Guide* (SSI/DoH, 1991, para. 4.2), may usefully be approached as a series of linked activities, which are to:

- determine the type of plan
- explore the resources of users and carers
- establish preferences
- cost the care plan
- agree service objectives
- coordinate the plan
- identify unmet need
- record the care plan.

The meaning and content of each of these activities will be explored in this and subsequent chapters. Reference will also be made to *Fair Access to Care Services* (FACS) (DoH, 2002g) which in para. 47 addresses key requirements of the care plan, with a narrower focus than the *Practitioners' Guide*. So FACS lists the six key requirements of the care plan in operational terms as:

- noting eligible needs and associated risks
- identifying preferred outcomes of service provision
- making contingency plans to manage emergency changes
- giving details of services to be provided and any charges the individual has been assessed to pay, or if direct payments have been agreed
- detailing contributions which users and carers and others are willing and able to make
- setting a review date.

Although this listing of activities is a template answer to the basic question of what should go into the care plan, it falls short of locating the care planning function within the parameters of social work. Social work intervention will focus on issues of risk, protection, support, therapy and empowerment; these are the major agendas of which care planning is derivative. Basic agreement first needs to be reached on the goals of intervention and the outcome measures which are to be used to determine whether or not those goals are being achieved. The values on which the care plan is based must also be explicit in promoting self-determination and working actively with individuals and groups to counter discrimination. A care plan is not simply a 'basket of goods and services; it is a complex set of human relationships', the achievement and maintenance of which require skills in both negotiation and the management of change (Smale and Tuson, 1993).

Determine the type of plan

All users in receipt of a continuing service should have a care plan (SSI/DoH, 1991, para. 4.3), even if the assessment of need is a simple one which can be met by a single service. Without a definition of objectives, even for a single service, the functions of monitoring and review become meaningless. One of the fundamental objectives of care management is to clarify the responsibilities of agencies (DoH, 1989b) and the care plan is an essential tool in locating such responsibilities. Who should receive a copy of the care plan? Clearly, all users and carers and significant service providers, although, as an example, Mencap (1995) found that a minority of users received copies of the care plan and the format was unhelpful. In particular, there was little scope for recording differences of opinion and emphasis between care managers, users of services and carers.

Explore the resources of users and carers

Consensus often appears to be assumed, where in reality there is none. The *Practitioners' Guide* (SSI/DoH, 1991, p. 67) recommends that points of difference between the user, carer, care planning practitioner or other agency should be contained in the care plan. FACS (DoH, 2002g, para. 47) refers simply to 'a note of the eligible needs and associated risks' as the first of six key requirements of the care plan. There is no exploration of how the different priorities of agencies, service users and carers fit with eligibility criteria definitions of acceptable risk and need, in particular in work with involuntary clients in mental health and the criminal justice system.

> Care planning should not be seen as matching needs with services 'off the shelf' but as an opportunity to rethink service provision for a particular individual. (SSI/DoH, 1991, para. 4.12)

This statement lies at the heart of individualised care planning. Separating the purchaser and providing functions ought in theory to free purchasers from conventional service provision and enable budgets to be used in creative ways. Early models of care management, where care managers were provided with sums of money equivalent to the cost of residential care to maintain people in the community, were based on this premise, although conservatism may be compounded by the inability of care managers to purchase outside lists of approved providers. In the design of service, at both a strategic and an individual level, user involvement is critical to the provision of a quality service but requires investment in terms of time, energy and commitment. The Shaping our Lives project commissioned by the Joseph Rowntree Foundation found that present systems were perceived as paternalistic and current practices around 'user involvement' were patchy and tokenistic, leading to 'involvement fatigue' (Turner et al., 2003).

Establish preferences

Arguably, from the inception of the new system of community care, considerations such as user choice were never designed to take precedence within care planning. In its report for the Department of Health, Price Waterhouse (1991, para. 10) envisaged that the purchaser/provider split would 'facilitate increased client choice through the empowerment of care managers' (not the empowerment of users). The report went on to say:

> It is important to remember that the empowerment of care managers on behalf of clients does not mean absolute client choice. Professional views, departmental policy, budgetary constraints and availability will all have a major impact on the package of care provided.

Operational and strategic imperatives may thus overcome both user choice and professional judgement. For example, cost efficiency in the provision of in-house daycare may make that a preferred option over use of the independent sector. Departmental policy may determine who gets what type of resource within those available even when assessment protocols require user preferences to be discussed.

Eligibility criteria

Eligibility criteria are used to target resources to those deemed to be most in need of them; 'need' being seen as a cost–benefit concept. The question of who should be in the target groups is based on the valuation of outputs, for example keeping people out of residential care. Prioritising need in this way has led to a reduction or non-availability of services for some people. As resources become more limited, so people with lesser needs may find that they no longer qualify for a service, or that a service previously provided, such as domestic help, is no longer available. Discretion also remains in how to meet needs. For example, the provision of residential care for someone who would otherwise need 24-hour care at home would be a proper use of discretion in the allocation of resources. However, rigid adherence to a policy that no more than a certain number of hours of home care would be provided at home would be an unlawful fettering of discretion. Given the individualised nature of assessments, each case would still have to be dealt with on its merits. FACS is designed to structure such local discretion in providing services following assessment according to the critical nature of individuals' needs, and to remove barriers to access that may have existed between, for example, services for older people and young adults with similar needs.

Commissioning and contracting

A systematic process for recording the provision of community-based services as a client-based system has been provided by the RAP (referrals, assessments and packages of care for adults) project (available at www.doh.gov.uk/rap/index.htm). In 2001–02, 71 per cent of community-based services (for example home care, daycare and meals) were received by people aged 75 or over. However, the number of households receiving services had fallen, whilst the intensity of home care packages had increased, thus showing increased targeting of resources. Average contact hours in 2001–02 were 8.1 per household, compared to 3.5 per household in 1993. The proportion of this provided by the independent sector had increased massively, from 5 per cent in 1993 to 64 per cent in 2002. The number of residential beds provided by the independent sector had also increased from 75 per cent of total provision in 1994 to 84 per cent in 2001. This means an increase in commissioning arrangements whatever services are provided, with associated transaction costs in negotiation and monitoring for the organisation and the care manager.

An inevitable tension is created between the economic and social objectives of care management; managing the budget versus advocacy for the best interests of the service user. Mares (1996) identifies a new range of business skills needed by care managers. These are handling contracts, costing care packages, negotiating prices with providers, monitoring the quality of service and sourcing suppliers. In addition, care managers should be aware of the 'cost' of their own time involved in such activities, as well as that of other professional colleagues such as occupational therapists or home care managers whose skills and resources they may wish to include in the assessment.

Local authorities employ three main types of contract (DoH, 1993a):

- *block contracts* – the purchaser buys access to a part or the whole of a service or facility for a specified price
- *cost or volume contracts* – a volume of service and a total cost is agreed and any additional service is provided on an individual price basis
- *individual or spot contracts* – the purchaser contracts for a service for an individual user for a specified time at an agreed price.

Each of these types of contract combines different risks for the provider, and varying degrees of flexibility for the user. Care managers need to know what type of contract is favoured by their local authority in what sort of circumstances.

Bamford (2001) describes how New Labour has replaced compulsory competitive tendering with best value regimes but with diversity and choice replaced by economy of scale. Thus the individual purchasing function has been subsumed into a broader commissioning role, with Bamford using the term 'micro-commissioning' to describe the process of developing a care package to meet the needs of the user. Care managers remain accountable, in purchasing decisions as elsewhere, for their professional judgement in making placements or providing services. Best value may not mean selecting the cheapest service, but balancing cost against the quality of service provided. Thus a key difference between traditional social work and care management is that the latter seeks out potential new resources and works out which will provide the best solution for the individual user within the budget available. Traditional social work, by contrast, involves coordinating existing services and liaising with other agencies.

Research into the process of care management in Scotland (Stalker and Campbell, 2002) showed how managerial control and a contract culture had taken a firm hold since earlier research by Stalker (1994) and Lapsley et al. (1994). In 1994, accepted social work measures such as client choice were prioritised over the objective analysis of efficiency and effectiveness, for example in the retention of relatively high-cost local authority care. By 2002, managerial restrictions on accessing service providers was more in evidence, but choice was also limited by the patchy availability of good quality private sector providers. Although budgets devolved to individual care managers were not widespread, where they did exist, they were not only seen as more empowering by staff, but they also made service delivery quicker and enabled contract compliance to be better monitored. It is probably still true that care budgets are hard to forecast: 'member thresholds' within local authorities may operate to underwrite budgets for particularly popular services and the boundaries with informal care are flexible to move costs (Lapsley, 1996). So, despite a higher profile for business skills and methods, financial rigour is inherently more difficult to achieve in a social care context.

Cost the care plan

Assessment and exploration of resources are stages in care management that should precede any assessment of the financial position of the service user. Thus the local authority should respond in an equitable way to need, irrespective of any contribution which may be sought to the cost of the services. For service users, however, the comparative cost of different options may be essential information in deciding whether they will, for example, opt for an intensive package of domiciliary care rather than a daycare option: 'Users should always know the estimated cost to themselves of any options under active consideration [and] no user should agree a care plan before they have been advised in writing of any charges involved' (SSI/DoH, 1991, paras 4.16 and 4.18). Similarly, FACS requires user contributions to be assessed for inclusion in the care plan. Details of benefit entitlements and charging policies are contained in Chapter 9.

Agree service objectives

What is the status of the care plan once it has been devised? The *Practitioners' Guide* (SSI/DoH, 1991, para. 4.38) puts forward the view that 'the care plan does not have a legal standing as a contract', although 'to reinforce the sense of commitment', contributors (including the user) may be asked to signify their agreement by signing. For the local authority's part, 'a care plan may be used as evidence in the consideration of a complaint'. Although it should be used to clarify service objectives, a care plan is not a document fixed in time, and should contain within itself some flexibility for minor adjustments to be made, a date for its own review (often six or eight weeks hence, depending on administrative practice) or a statement of the contingency factors which would trigger an earlier review.

The basic question to ask is whether the service has been effective, in the sense of achieving its objectives, such as retention in the community or a problem-free discharge from hospital. Describing social care services in terms of inputs, process, outputs and outcomes is an approach which has been adapted from business management. The advantage of specifying services in these terms is that it enables service planners to analyse more closely the way in which particular services achieve results (Mares, 1996). The importance of outcome measures and difficulties in their definition are further examined in Chapter 6. Review enables authorities to check that objectives are still relevant and are being achieved. There are practical difficulties, of course, in breaking continuity by allocating different functions to different personnel, particularly where review staff may be less well qualified than assessors, and providers may have a financial interest in continuing services. More fundamental, however, is the presumption (or so it seems) in favour of short-term rather than long-term involvement by assessors and purchasers of service. Some of the dynamic nature of assessments must inevitably be lost in this process, and the opportunity for methods of intervention such as the psychodynamic, which are based on a continuing and evolving relationship with the client, are lost (Coulshed, 1991). The problem has been particularly noted in mental health services (Huxley, 1993).

Coordinate the plan

The coordination and implementation of the care plan is the fifth stage of care management; 'the guiding principle of implementation should be to achieve the stated objectives of the care plan with the minimum intervention possible' (SSI/DoH, 1991, para. 5.1). Minimum intervention is defined, however, not in terms of values, such as self-determination and empowerment, but in utilitarian terms minimising the number of service providers involved. The example given is of introducing 'generic care workers who perform a range of tasks that have traditionally been divided between home care and auxiliary nursing staff' (SSI/ DoH, 1991, para. 5.1). This certainly has been a feature of some care management projects, most notably Darlington (Challis et al., 1995), and is a feature of partnership agendas; but is in itself not uncontentious, given that healthcare is that which is provided free at the point of delivery, although social care has to be paid for by financial assessment.

Implementation is viewed solely in terms of securing the necessary resources or services, not in terms of targeting change within systems. The radical perspective on personal issues as consequences of structural deficits cannot be accommodated within this definition of implementation. The care plan is viewed as a closed system, individualistic in nature. The preferred role for the practitioner is that of social care planner, not service broker. In some case, of course, the agency may be seeking to impose a service that the user does not want but which is deemed necessary for his or her protection or to monitor her or his progress – supervised discharge from psychiatric care is a case in point. Where legislation imposes protective duties on the local authority, tension will inevitably exist between client empowerment and professional accountability.

Services contributing to a package of care may be nothing more than a listing of conventional service provision. Kathryn Ellis (1993), in her research into user and carer participation in needs assessment, was continually struck by how marginal the support provided by social services or any other community-based services was to most people's lives. By framing people's experience solely in terms of the limited context of community care, their aspirations about overall lifestyle are not considered, and an opportunity has been lost for the definitions of need used in assessment to be used to encompass a broader slice of people's lives (Ellis, 1993, p. 41). This should be what 'negotiating the scope of assessment' really means, if as the guidance says, 'the individual's needs are to seen in their proper social context' (SSI/DoH, 1991, para. 3.3). Certainly, for a comprehensive assessment, the *Practitioners' Guide* (SSI/DoH, 1991, p. 58) suggests that the following issues are covered: self-perceived needs; abilities, attitudes and lifestyle; race and culture; social network and support; housing; finance; transport; and risk. Similarly, FACS identifies needs and risks in relation to social roles, including roles as parent and employee, as defining eligibility for services as clearly as physical needs. One would expect, then, that care plans would mirror such agendas.

In the provision of resources to meet needs identified in the care plan, authorities should be free to use a variety of providers and not be constrained by conventional patterns of service organisation. This is what needs-led assessment really means. So a need for social stimulation will not necessarily be met by a day centre place; it may be met by the provision of transport and a facilitator to enable someone to visit family or friends. Prior to the introduction of community care, there used to be difficulties with 'out of authority' placements that local authorities would not fund. With the opening up of markets in social care, this should no longer be a barrier; indeed it may be maladministration not to make use of such flexibility in service provision.

Identify unmet need

Care management was conceived as a cyclical process (see Figure 1.1) in which feedback from the user of services was incorporated back into the planning stage. Success in this process means knowing how to identify, and what to do about, unmet need. Para. 4.33 of the *Practitioners' Guide* (SSI/DoH, 1991) sees a benefit in differentiating between types of unmet need, including those that are:

- *statutory obligations*, for example those included in the Disabled Persons Act 1986
- defined as *entitlements* under local policies, for example failure to provide services within defined timescales
- *current policies or criteria*, for example the emerging needs of those with HIV/AIDS.

The consequences of failing to meet these categories of need will undoubtedly be different. The identification of new needs must be considered when service development plans are revised. Failure to achieve internal targets, or those devised externally, for example performance indicators set by the Department of Health, will attract the attention of local authorities' senior management, while failure to fulfil statutory obligations is both a major cause for concern at an organisational level, as well as being open to challenge by individuals through litigation (see Chapter 6).

There may well be a clash of perspectives even within legislation. In *R (A&B) v. East Sussex County Council (No. 2)* (reported in Clements, 2004), the courts were asked to decide how local authorities should resolve the different interests of two profoundly disabled sisters to be lifted safely with dignity, and the interests of their paid carers to a safe system of work within guidance from the Health and Safety Executive (HSE). The local authority had accepted that its 'no manual handling' policy was unlawful, but the court had to find a balance between the rights of people to independence and social integration and the avoidance of unacceptable risk to carers. The balance would be different in every case, but may require the installation of specialist equipment beyond that usually supplied in the community. What would not be acceptable, and therefore negligent, would be for the authority to allow an untrained family carer to carry out tasks deemed too dangerous for its own employees.

Record the care plan

Doel and Shardlow (1998) identify four specific purposes behind recording information. These are: procedural; investigative and speculative; personal; and providing continuity. As far as care plans are concerned, the procedural aspect – providing an accessible account of past processes and agreements – is uppermost. The investigative and speculative function of recording will be important when complex situations are being explored, as in cases of suspected abuse. The personal aspect of recording underlines the value of life history and is linked to client access to files. Both this and the function of records in ensuring continuity of care are important in long-term work. The translation of care plans drawn up by care managers in the community into care plans within daycare and residential care has not been much considered. As an example of good practice in this area, Reed and Stanley (2003) describe a practice development project that produced a user-led daily living plan to facilitate communication of the daily living preferences of older people. The plan sought to ensure that continuity of care could be maintained when the older person moved from hospital to a care home and made evaluation of outcomes more transparent.

Social work interventions: risk and protection; support and care

The social worker as care manager will, by virtue of his or her professional role, be involved in the social work agendas of risk and protection as well as support and care. The care plan will be an important tool in risk assessment and risk management. Organisational constraints on purchasers may limit opportunities for further direct work to be undertaken with individuals once tasks have been identified for action within the care plan. Longer term therapeutic involvement may be seen as a provider service to be bought in, rather than as part of a holistic process. The relevance of both risk assessment and protection, and support and care, to the process of care planning is discussed below.

Risk and protection

Stalker (2003) identifies risk as a major, if not overarching, preoccupation in social work. Theories range from a scientific approach to risk, in terms of the probability of events happening, to social constructionist approaches of harm focusing on perceptions rather than realities. Social models of risk, looking at environmental factors such as poverty and poor housing, are not well developed. Kemshall et al. (1997) argue that social work's concern with risk as uncertainty is based on a loss of faith in knowledge and traditional power hierarchies in post-modern societies. But Stalker (2003, p. 221) considers the absence of a contribution from the people using services as 'a glaring omission' – those who are perceived by professionals as being at risk or posing a risk to others.

Many commentators argue that risk management is increasingly taking the form of risk avoidance, located at the controlling end of the continuum (Stalker, 2003). This approach uses risk as a forensic rather than a predictive device; a means of allocating blame once something has gone wrong. An example of both approaches is provided by the NHS policy on risk management and organisational controls (DoH, 2000). Within this document, risk identification is seen as both proactive (in terms of prediction) and retrospective (avoiding reoccurrence). The prioritisation of risks within a risk register is designed to create a manageable programme of risk targets. Residual risk, which cannot be controlled, is shared amongst the health community through the 'clinical negligence scheme for trusts', operated by the NHS Litigation Authority. Control over individual practice is sought by the systematic recording of the process and outcome of assessment and decision-making and the evidence base of reasons for the decision. Fear of being blamed is heightened by adverse media coverage, the threat of litigation or public inquiries (Stalker, 2003); the consequence of which is defensive practice (Banks, 2002). Bamford (2001, p. 118) presciently comments that the Bristol children's heart surgery inquiry, in which risky professional decisions were effectively unchallengeable, may mark a watershed in shifting the hands-off approach of commissioners on professional issues, as they feel increasingly responsible morally as well as legally for the quality of the service that is delivered.

Risk analysis

Risk analysis in an actuarial sense involves both the estimation and evaluation of risk. Estimation includes statistical incidence (it is known, for example, that 1 in 5 of the population over the age of 80 will suffer from dementia) and the application of general knowledge to particular situations (for example the combustible qualities of domestic gas). The evaluation of risk is, however, a balancing process, in which the application of judgement is bought to bear. The factors to be taken into account are:

- the likelihood of a particular event happening
- the reasonably foreseeable consequences of that event happening
- the interests of the people affected by the consequences of the event happening
- the cost of taking precautions against the happening of the event or its consequences
- duties owed by other people.

'Is he at risk?' is a question often posed in a range of different circumstances. It may be asked, for example, in relation to people with dementia who forget to light their gas fire when they turn it on, so 'running the risk' of explosion and hypothermia. It may also be used, say, of a person with learning disabilities living alone, who is finding it difficult to say 'no' to local people who want to borrow and use his or her home for their convenience. The risks for each must be particularised, but the general issues are the same as those of risk assessment and risk management. Doel and Shardlow (1998) analyse risk in social work practice as an amalgam of the perceived dangerousness of the situation, and the social worker's willingness to intervene. It cannot be assumed that the former necessarily leads to the latter. Mediating factors for social workers may be:

- attitudes to taking control
- cultural views about acceptable behaviour
- fear of making mistakes
- fears about their own safety
- beliefs about the role of social work in society
- confidence about their professional judgement
- knowledge about the legal context of social work practice.

These factors create moral dilemmas for managers as well as practitioners (Dawson and Butler, 2003). Although the CA 1989 quantifies risk in terms of significant harm as the threshold for statutory involvement, there is no exact equivalent in adult care. Nor are there complex procedural arrangements for

assessing risk, allocating and authorising responsibility and monitoring intervention, such as exist in child protection procedures. The only exception to this in
adult care is the introduction of supervision registers and supervised discharge
arrangements under mental health legislation (see Chapter 10) and the
proceduralisation of adult protection in guidance (see below). This has the effect
of leaving individual practitioners exposed, and individual clients without formal
means of involvement in decision-making.

So, taking as an example the person with dementia who forgets to light the gas
fire, the likelihood of an explosion happening is high, but the likelihood of the
person suffering damage from the cold would depend on the time of year. The
consequences of an explosion would be grave not only for the person him/herself
but also for his/her neighbours. However, if the risk were only one of
hypothermia, the consequences would affect only the individual him/herself
and might well be dependent on his/her general state of health. The cost in
practical terms of taking precautions against the event happening could involve a
change in the form of heating in the house to a safer central heating system, or
disconnection of the gas supply whilst the householder was alone in the house. No
doubt there would be some discussion of whether the individual was safe to
remain at home or whether residential care should be considered.

An often forgotten element in the equation is the emotional cost of leaving a
familiar environment, but is one which should be weighed in the balance. The
analysis of risk is often carried out so as to avoid criticism if something goes
wrong which public authorities know about. Is this sufficient reason for
overriding self-determination? The answer depends on whether or not there is a
duty to intervene; the only duty under s.47 NHSCCA 1990 is to assess for
community care services, not a duty to 'make safe'; outside the Mental Health Act
1983 and section 47 of the National Assistance Act 1947, there are no grounds for
intervention if services are refused (McDonald, 2004). In the case of the person
with dementia, the client's perception of the risk is important; is he/she able to
evaluate what is happening and make an informed decision if it is a situation
he/she wishes to continue to live with. Is the social worker comfortable or not
with the use of authority?

Much will then depend on the management of the risk. Interventions may be
devised to manage the risk by introducing assistance into the home, or providing
other forms of support. Advocacy services may be helpful in monitoring
satisfaction with the intervention. Above all, in risk management, administrative
systems are necessary to provide a forum for decision-making and enable review
to happen. Preferably these should be interagency; as with care management
generally, unintended conflicts can arise if there are different agency strategies for
dealing with the risks associated with vulnerable clients.

Support and care and the social work role

Prior to the implementation of the NHSCCA 1990, there was disquiet that social
work skills in intervention were being overlooked within the process of care
planning. Concentration on the purchasing function is acknowledged to have had
this effect (DoH, 1993, para. 47):

The provision of advice and on-going support for clients by social workers is very important in professional terms. However, the language of care management can lead to this function being under emphasised as compared to brokering for the provision of services by third parties.

The assumption that the difficulties of vulnerable people can be resolved within a brief timescale is clearly false. If continuing support is not given, then re-referral is inevitable for at least a proportion of these cases.

The American system of case management, on which care management is based, was never seen as a short-term solution; it was always seen as a procedure for dealing with long-term cases, within which a combination of practical assistance, therapy and support could be offered. The prominence of the task-centred method of social work within care management may have been misconstrued to favour short-term involvement, and based on only practical concerns. Yet there is clearly a place for the task-centred approach within long-term work in which issues may be dealt with sequentially; and it is a misrepresentation of the term 'task-centred' to see it as irrelevant to emotional or relationship problems. The role of the social worker can be as confidant, therapist, broker, advocate or any combination of these, as a means to implement the care plan and effect change (Goldberg and Warburton, 1979).

Clearly, these different ends will attract different strategies. Major environmental change may require negotiation with other agencies, such as housing, to physically relocate an individual. But even in such a situation, skill as a negotiator will not be all that is needed; sensitivity to a feeling of loss for the old environment may invoke the use of counselling skills until the adaptation is made. Changes in the personal/social environment may need the use of groupwork skills to integrate people into a new social environment such as a day centre. Changes in social roles will involve people in transitions; to worker, to parent, to carer, for example. Changes in behaviour and attitude, including offending, may be amenable to a behaviourist or cognitive approach, and work with relationships may involve family counselling, family work or family therapy. The orientation of the worker and his or her reading of the situation will influence the choice of method, but the range of interventions available illustrates the complexities within the care planning role.

The role played by the social work practitioner will itself need to be adapted for different organisational contexts. Hughes (1995), adapting Øvretveit (1993), describes four roles which practitioners may undertake in different situations:

- the care profession – specific role
- the role as member of the care package team
- the care manager role
- the role of the developer of services.

The 'care profession – specific role' describes the situation in which the practitioner is a caseworker, having responsibility for the assessment and provision of professional help, with the role and function vis-à-vis other professionals being one of liaison rather than coordination. The member of the care package team will provide profession-specific services but in the context of a multidisciplinary network of service providers directly accountable to the care manager for their own role within a package of care. The care manager may or may not be providing a profession-specific service but is responsible as manager for orchestrating, maintaining, monitoring and reviewing the effectiveness of the care package (Renshaw, 1988). The practitioner as developer of services has á role to play in stimulating agencies through the commissioning process to provide what is in short supply or lacking. These are the tasks that have to be performed in order to deliver services effectively. How can they be achieved by practitioners?

An example of the professional-specific role might be a social worker in a hospital setting, whereas the social worker as member of a care package team may be working within a community mental health team or community learning disability team. So far, so good. In relation to the care manager, however, will it in fact be possible to divorce that role from the professional qualification of the post holder? Arguably the skills, knowledge and values of the social work practitioner will not stand alone, but will become enmeshed, as described above, in the role of care manager (Reigate, 1995; Sheppard, 1995). The practitioner as developer of services is an interesting role. Certainly in that role, as described, there will be a responsibility to use information on unmet need to stimulate new services, and this could apply to in-house services, such as domiciliary care, in equal measure. There will also be a need to explore community networks proactively: 'Entrepreneurial case management requires the mobilisation, indeed the creation of informal networks, not merely their support or revival' (Davies and Challis, 1986, p. 47). This is akin to a community development role. There is also another developmental role to be undertaken; with the concentration of qualified workers on the purchasing side, provider side workers may need additional support and input in dealing with more complex cases and so a consultative function may arise and may need to be incorporated into the care plan. Thus care management can expand the traditional client-focused role of social work into more diverse and collective activities even within an individual care plan.

Abuse and protection

The greater concentration of vulnerable people in the community has awakened awareness of the potential for abuse and a desire to explore means of protection from exploitation and neglect. The focus of such concern has historically been the abuse of elderly people, but not exclusively so (ADSS, 1991); the abuse, particularly sexual abuse, of people with learning disabilities is of increasing concern (Brown and Turk, 1992; Williams and Evans, 2000). Parallels may be drawn with experience of domestic violence and child abuse in particular (Stevenson, 1996).

Adult abuse is a socially constructed phenomenon, insofar as various aspects of behaviour and their consequences are defined by others as constituting or not constituting a category which is given the title 'abuse'. Various definitions may exist which focus on the legality of the action, the intention with which it was performed or its consequence. The definition adopted by Action on Elder Abuse, an organisation prominent in this field, locates abuse within the context of caring relationships, and defines as abusive, actions which may not be illegal; it also covers inaction (or neglect) as well as action: 'Elder abuse is a single or repeated act or lack of appropriate action occurring within any relationship where there is an expectation of trust which causes harm or distress to an older person' (Action on Elder Abuse, 1996). Five main types of abuse are detailed:

- *physical* – for example hitting, slapping, burning, pushing, restraining or giving too much medication or the wrong medication
- *psychological* – for example shouting, swearing, frightening, blaming, ignoring or humiliating a person
- *financial* – for example the illegal or unauthorised use of a person's property, money or other valuables
- *sexual* – for example forcing a person to take part in sexual activity without consent
- *neglect* – for example where a person is deprived of food, heat, clothing, comfort or essential medication.

These types of abuse may be distinct or may be experienced at the same time. Mutually abusive situations, for example between an older person and their spouse or child, may well exist and it is accepted that older people may themselves abuse people who care for them.

Prevalence and incidence

The hidden nature of abuse makes reporting highly variable and is bound up with social awareness generally and definitions and categories of abuse. In the UK, unlike the USA, there are no mandatory reporting laws for professionals to report abuse. The only study of prevalence in the UK was undertaken by Ogg and Bennett (1992), which produced figures of a prevalence of 15.2 for physical abuse per 1,000 population and 53.9 for verbal abuse. Financial abuse also had a prevalence of 15.2. Surveys amongst more vulnerable groups of people have given much higher numbers; the best known of these is Homer and Gilleard's (1990) study of 51 carers of patients receiving respite care in hospital, 45 of whom admitted to some form of abuse.

Although victims of abuse are found across the whole age spectrum, irrespective of social class, gender or ethnic origin, there is evidence that they are disproportionately in the older age groups and more likely to be female. Cultural factors may also have an influence on the type and nature of abuse (since physical abuse is more highly correlated with living in the same household and male abusers). Financial abuse is spread across the income range to a greater extent than physical or psychological abuse; people living on their own are also at greater risk of financial abuse and neglect by others (McCreadie, 1996).

Social and professional abuse

There have, however, been critics of the adoption of this campaign by professionals, given that there is little direct evidence that older people themselves see abuse by carers as a major concern (Biggs, 1997). Their concern is about standards of care in domiciliary and residential services and lack of the basic necessities of life, in terms of adequate income and responsive services (Robertson, 1995). Refocusing attention on abuse within a domestic setting may paradoxically assist the redefinition of abuse in residential care as an issue of 'quality' or service neglect, rather than a matter for criminal law or disciplinary procedures. Seeing abuse as an aspect of interpersonal relationships also excludes abuse which is rooted in ageism, racism or sexism, and thus makes these issues more difficult to challenge directly.

The service response

Service responses need to be set in the context of an assessment of the need for community care services as a whole, within which abuse is one particular issue (ADSS, 1995). Stevenson (1996) expresses concern about the proceduralisation of adult abuse in the same way that procedures have come to dominate child protection, although she sees some proceduralisation as necessary to ensure interagency cooperation. No procedures however can compensate for professional awareness of the nature of abuse and appropriate responses. The response chosen will depend on the analysis of the causes of abuse. It is clear that not all these analyses fit the dependent victim/stressed carer model, there being no evidence that the stress of caring in itself precipitates abuse.

Homer and Gilleard (1990) indicated that different types of abuse could be ascribed to different causes and there was no one correct approach to interpretation or intervention:

> Physical abuse is perpetrated by people with disturbed and disorganised personalities irrespective of the physical and mental state of the abused ... Verbal abuse and neglect were both significantly related to poor pre-morbid relationships, an association not seen for physical abuse ... neglect was associated with socially dysfunctional carers. (Homer and Gilleard, 1990, cited in McCreadie, 1996, p. 34)

Decalmer and Glendenning (1997) propose a number of models for understanding abuse, which can be free of professional bias and the basis on which crisis intervention and prevention techniques are developed:

- *The situational model*: based on an amalgam of structural factors such as low income and isolation and factors personal to the abused person, such as poor health, physical dependency and carer stress or burnout.
- *Social exchange theory*: based on the idea that social interaction involves a balance of rewards and punishments which are upset by the dependency of the older person and the greater powerfulness of the carer.
- *Symbolic interactionism*: referring to the adoption over time of familiar roles and expectations. These may be upset when one person unexpectedly becomes a carer or a strong parent declines in cognitive ability because of dementia.

- *Personal characteristics of abusers and victims*: emphasis here is on the psychopathology of the abuser (related to mental health, drug or alcohol dependency) and their social isolation. A history of violence may also be a factor, as may the quality of the relationship between the abuser and the abused.

Any of the above may be considered to be risk factors of abuse, but there is insufficient evidence from research to suggest that any of them are of predictive value. What is important is that the individual worker is aware of his/her own perspective on the situation and where it comes from. Interviewing skills are of primary importance:

> Familiarity with interviewing people in a non-directive fashion about sensitive issues, being able to tolerate ambiguity and use counselling skills are necessary prerequisites to assessment and intervention in this area, as is an awareness of how our own personal values and beliefs about ageing and abuse can affect our judgement – not always in the best interests of the abused, client or patient. (Goudie and Alcott, 1994, p. 235)

The law provides an insufficient framework to allow for intervention (McDonald, 1993; ADSS, 1995; Law Commission, 1995). In adult care there is no equivalent of the emergency protection order or child assessment order provided under the CA 1989, nor is there any power (outside the Mental Health Act 1983) to secure entry to premises, if entry is refused. Section 47 of the National Assistance Act 1948 is an anachronistic piece of legislation which provides for the compulsory removal from home of people who are chronically sick or aged and living in insanitary conditions who are not in receipt of proper care. It may be used in cases of neglect (including self-neglect), but has been much criticised as draconian and procedurally deficient (application is made to the magistrates' court and no legal aid is available) (McDonald, 2004).

Although there has been no significant legal change, the publication of policy guidance *No Secrets* (DoH, 2000c) on interagency cooperation in the protection of vulnerable adults has marked an important formalisation of issues relating to protection in adult care. The term 'vulnerable adults' cuts across conventional user group divides to encompass older people, people with disabilities and those with mental health problems. Indeed, any person in need of community care services who is unable to protect themselves from harm or exploitation may be seen as a vulnerable adult. 'Vulnerable adult' is a term which is also used in the Mental Capacity Act 2004 (see Chapter 8) and, although it has connotations of passivity and dependency, it is intended to reflect an inclusive approach to assessment and service provision which is usable across agencies. The guidance defines abuse in wide terms as interference with a person's personal and human rights, and extends the Action on Elder Abuse definition by including institutional and discriminatory abuse. Although social services authorities are the lead agency under *No Secrets*, cases in which there is an initial allegation of criminal activity are to be referred to the police for investigation. For the first time, the Youth Justice and Criminal Evidence Act 1999 has enabled vulnerable adults to be interviewed on video and have protection in court similar to that accorded to child witnesses. Conceptually, the protection of adult abuse procedures has developed, with the inclusion of institutional abuse on the list of types of abuse that will attract protection, and the focus is also extended beyond the domestic sphere to abuse by persons in the community.

Although *No Secrets* (DoH, 2000c) provides a national framework for the development of local policies, guidance for practitioners will continue to be variable. Research by Preston-Shoot and Wigley (2000) found that there was scope for improvement in interagency work concerning agreed definitions and responsibility for carrying out protection plans. The absence of housing providers from multiagency arrangements also contributed to a lack of choice when moving individuals out of abusive situations; invariably it was the older person who had to move. Social workers were also not given guidance on how to respond if people did not want action taken and privileged self-determination over protection, without setting the initial rejection of help in the context of exploitation or intimidation. The importance of providing continuing support to victims of abuse is identified by Pritchard (2000); many older people who have been abused will have complex stories to tell and will need assistance beyond the stages of investigation and disclosure. It appears that there is still a need for raising awareness of the prevalence of abuse, taking evidence particularly from research into older people (Preston-Shoot and Wigley, 2000) and people with learning difficulties (Williams and Evans, 2000). There is still a substantial process of denial concerning abuse; non-specialist services may not recognise the extent to which they have vulnerable clients, and dealing with 'crime' rather than 'welfare' is a rare experience for care professionals.

Reform of the law is long overdue, despite the recommendation of the Law Commission (1995) that 'a new jurisdiction' (or court, akin to the court of protection) is needed to deal with both personal issues and financial protection (see Chapter 9). This new jurisdiction, according to the Law Commission, would apply to people who were mentally incapacitated, that is, unable to make decisions for themselves because of mental disorder or learning disabilities, and would provide a forum in which conflicts over care or access could be decided. An expansion of the scope of powers of attorney is also proposed to enable people to appoint attorneys to take decisions on their behalf concerning, for example, admission to residential care or medical treatment. This would clarify and formalise the position of family and carers who are often called upon to make such decisions without clear legal authority. The Mental Capacity Act 2004, which would give effect to the Law Commission's recommendations, proposes reform of the law through lasting powers of attorney and advance directives, although it contains no formal duty to investigate allegations of abuse as a matter of public law.

Using the concept of significant harm, borrowed from the CA 1989, as a threshold of intervention would enable multidisciplinary assessments of physical, psychological and emotional harm to be made (McDonald, 1993). The criteria for intervention should follow the 'essential powers' approach of guardianship under the Mental Health Act 1983, that is, the minimum necessary intervention (Hoggett, 1989). Such intervention would be the 'legislative mandate' that Marsh and Fisher (1992) look for as a basis for partnership where consent cannot be given. If guardianship is the model to be followed, these essential powers would specify where that person was required to live, medical attendance to be given and monitoring visits to be permitted. In child protection, it has also been shown that collaborative work is less effective after investigation, in relation to the 'protection plan'; the implications of this finding will need to be considered in the protection of adults (Stevenson, 1996). Consideration should also be given to prioritise vulnerable adults whose proper health and development will be jeopardised without the provision of services for them by the local authority, much as children may be defined as 'in need' within the Children Act.

Concluding comments

This chapter looked at the process of care planning against the requirements of best value in the provision of publicly funded services and the types of contract that agencies can enter into for the commissioning of social care. These technical processes are contrasted with the continuing professional agendas of providing support and protection to vulnerable individuals. The assessment of risk is a central skill in social work and sits alongside the recognition of new responsibilities to respond to exploitation and abuse as well as to support the choices made by service users. When services have been put in place, it cannot be assumed that needs will not change or innovations become available. Monitoring the effectiveness of the care package and reviewing its continued relevance, with a view to making changes if necessary, are the important final two stages of the system of care management. This also presents an opportunity for unmet need to be recorded and fed back into the care planning system. Chapter 5 looks in detail at the processes of monitoring and review and also examines the concepts of evaluation and effectiveness. A conventional package of care for vulnerable adults will contain elements of home support services, day services and possibly residential provision. These three areas of service delivery are separately examined in the light of policy and research, and in the application of key roles 2 and 3 of the National Occupational Standards concerning the reviewing and advocacy functions of social work.

PAUSE AND REFLECT

Find out what services are available locally for supporting service users in their own home. Relevant sources may be the statutory sector, voluntary sector or private providers. Services may include domiciliary care, befriending schemes or recreational activities. You may wish to focus on one particular group of people such as older people, carers or people recently discharged from hospital. Information thus gathered could be put together in the form of a reference book to assist in care planning. To what extent are these services based on 'ordinary life' principles that enable service users to participate in activities alongside other members of the community?

CASE STUDY

Adult protection

Helen Jones is 58 years old and has Parkinson's disease. She lives with her husband Tom who has taken early retirement. Tom helps Helen with washing and dressing and other aspects of personal care. They have no immediate family and live in a small village, five miles from the nearest town. Helen has been attending a voluntary sector day centre in the town two days a week for the last six months. Helen does not join in many of the activities at the day centre and has told staff that she would rather be at home. Her husband, however, has said that this is the only time he has to himself or to pursue his own hobbies. One day when Helen attends the day centre, staff notice bruising on the side of her face and behind her ear. When this is commented on, Helen breaks down in tears, saying that her husband has hit her for being too slow in getting ready to go out. He frequently handles her roughly and shouts at her. 'Please don't say anything though', says Helen, 'because he's told me that I will have to go into a home if I complain.'

If you were the manager of the day centre, how would you respond to this situation?

FURTHER READING

Bamford, T. (2001) *Commissioning and Purchasing*. London: Routledge/Community Care. A practical book which explains the differences between commissioning and purchasing decisions and explains the use made of different types of contract in social care. Clearly explained with exercises and case studies.

Glendinning, C., Powell, M. and Rummery, K. (eds) (2002) *Partnerships: New Labour and the Governance of Welfare*. Bristol: Policy Press.
An edited book exploring the change from a 'contract culture' to a 'partnership culture' across health and social care, education and the criminal justice system.

Kemshall, H. (2002) *Risk, Social Policy and Welfare*. Buckingham: Open University Press. Explores the transition from need to risk as the key organising principle of social policy. Includes chapters on developments in health policy, elder abuse and mental health.

CHAPTER 5

Monitoring and Review

Introduction

This chapter examines the processes of monitoring and review and looks at the recent research on evaluation and effectiveness. It examines the extent to which community care has made a real difference to people's lives. A range of services from daycare to domiciliary and residential care are examined as part of a continuum of services. The focus within monitoring and review should be on the provision of services which are effective to meet a range of different needs, and not simply an endorsement of established service provision. The following key roles are particularly evidenced in this chapter.

KEY ROLE 2

Plan, carry out, review and evaluate social work practice with individuals, families, carers, groups and communities and other professionals

KEY ROLE 3

Support individuals to represent their needs, views and circumstances

The production of welfare

The evaluation of outcomes, monitoring and review are essential components of the 'production of welfare' approach to care management, exemplified by early research into community care in Kent and elsewhere (Payne, 1995) and more recently by the Department of Health's *Outcomes of Social Care for Adults* research (Henwood and Waddington, 2002). The successful evaluation of outcomes depends on the clarity of objectives at the care planning stage, where clear goals are specified and strategic plans are worked out in order to achieve those goals. The monitoring process will then check that services are on target to meet those objectives. A review, however, is an opportunity for change, by allowing participants to stand back and reconsider what those goals should be and adjusting interim plans accordingly. If a mechanistic approach is taken to case monitoring and review, the complexities of relationships involved in supporting people in the community can become stereotypical. Short-term pragmatic issues will also tend to predominate over long-term aspirations. *Searching for Service* (SSI/DoH, 1996a) identified this at an early stage as a particular problem for young people with a learning disability, where 'getting through the week' took precedence over the longer term evaluation of educational and social needs in service planning. FACS (DoH, 2002g) now guides assessors to identify longer term as well as presenting needs. Proper monitoring and review means that care packages should be reviewed as a whole and not, as they have often been, by way of separate reviews, for example in residential care and daycare.

Monitoring

The *Managers' Guide* (SSI/DoH, 1991a, para. 2.29) makes it clear that systems of monitoring (and review) need not involve formal meetings, but can be undertaken in writing or by telephone. However, the important principle (para. 2.30) is that, wherever possible, monitoring and reviewing should be undertaken by someone who does not have a direct stake in the services provided. This is designed in principle to enable quality issues to be effectively addressed and services to remain needs-led.

Some service users may move in and out of the system. In mental health services, the CPA is predicated on the importance of regular monitoring and review of needs on a multidisciplinary basis. Huxley (1993) regards care management as failing people with long-term but fluctuating needs, if based on an inappropriate administrative rather than clinical model of care management. In the clinical model, direct face-to-face work is undertaken by the case manager, which is not only more effective therapeutically, but also enables continuous monitoring of relapses to take place. Nor does care management have to conform to short-term task-centred models. In the US, Raiff and Shore (1993) discuss involving family members as active partners in monitoring services and proactive 'case management extenders' in pulling in other resources. With regard to the monitoring function, consumers and family members should be specifically asked if they think that services are making a difference, what they would like the next steps to be and whether they are at this time feeling overinvolved and burdened. The opportunity should also be taken to provide up-to-date information about new resources and issues. The valuable interventions are those that build on family strengths rather than correcting deficits, and those that support family decisions and consciously attribute successful outcomes to the family's, rather than the case manager's, efforts (Raiff and Shore, 1993).

Review

Statutory reviews are familiar processes to social workers in childcare, and intervals between reviews are fixed by regulations in the case of children looked after by the local authority. Reviews may be presented as important decision-making occasions, but Thoburn (1986) challenges the view that a review is predominantly a decision-making occasion, pointing out that it is often the 'small' decisions made in the intervals between reviews that alter the outcome of a case. The issue may be whether, for example, to spend money on supporting visits by the family, or to extend the child's network by involving other significant persons in the community. Reviews in community care are not statutory; there is nothing in the NHSCCA 1990 that requires reviews to be held. There has, however, been an administrative tradition of holding reviews for separate services such as daycare and domiciliary care. As the *Managers' Guide* admits (SSI/DoH, 1991a, para. 2.30), in the past reviews have been accorded a low priority, so have either not taken place or been subject to considerable delay. Preliminary findings from SSI (1993a) inspections of community care services referred to the 'review time bomb', as energies have been focused on assessment, rather than review. This can mean that services are being provided where there is no longer a need, or are not adapting to changed circumstances.

What happens in practice?

There is evidence that in practice the tasks of monitoring and review are sometimes confused, particularly to the detriment of the monitoring task. Mencap's (1995) survey of service provision under community care noted the absence of clear local authority strategies for monitoring and attributed this partly to a paucity of government guidance on the issue. Only two out of thirty carers said that their care manager had told them about monitoring or how it is applied. Sometimes monitoring was substituted by review, with little opportunity to discuss or alter service provision in the interim.

The purchaser/provider split may have attenuated the withdrawal of assessors from the monitoring task. An example of inadequate monitoring of a care plan, exacerbated by the purchaser's withdrawal from responsibility for this task, is seen in a report from the local government ombudsman which led to a finding of maladministration against Newham Borough Council. In this case a disabled woman with complex and rapidly changing needs was allocated predominantly a home care service for both cleaning and personal care. Once the original care plan was agreed, responsibility for monitoring was put on the provider team which, because it was a provider team, had difficulty accessing the assessment team when the care plan began to break down. It also appears that insufficient flexibility was built into the original plan to deal with contingencies such as the complainant suffering further ligament injury and needing additional care. The care manager was also not readily available to respond to queries from home care assistants about the tasks included in the care plan, and was not aware that the service received was sometimes erratic.

Close liaison between care managers and home carers who are closest to the day-to-day issues is easily lost if lines of communication are cut by the purchaser/ provider split. It is also difficult to monitor a total package of care if provision is divided amongst a number of agencies. Evidence from Age Concern, Scotland (Robertson, 1995) and Sinclair et al. (2003) is that service users are keenly aware of the intimate and detailed knowledge that domiciliary workers have about their circumstances and wish this information to be fed back directly into care management systems.

Termination

Termination of social work involvement or a particular service is an issue not much dealt with in the literature; more attention has traditionally been focused on beginnings rather than endings. Raiff and Shore (1993, p. 60) acknowledge that:

> planned termination of advanced case management services to targeted high-risk clients is often an ethically and politically difficult decision, implying a judgement that a client's gains have been maximised or that a prediction of risk warrants this decision.

A number of other reasons for termination are identified, including de facto drop-out, client requests for termination or the tactical use of termination by the worker to precipitate a crisis that will re-engage 'uncooperative' clients.

More generally, the process of disengagement includes follow-up to ensure that a smooth transition is experienced and achieved goals can be sustained, leaving the door open to possible return if a change of circumstances should occur. Making a more effective or expanded use of available networks is often a precursor of termination of involvement with formal services. This shows the value respectively of being clear at the outset about the limits of involvement and the nature of the relationship. It also requires a criterion for success, or at least adequate progress, to be fixed at the outset; something which is fundamental to the partnership and which enhances self-esteem and confidence in the service user (Marsh and Fisher, 1992).

Evaluation and effectiveness

How do we know that the work we do and the services we provide are worthwhile? It may be possible to measure the effectiveness of a service in achieving a certain outcome, whether that is an older person remaining in the community rather than moving into residential care, or the achievement of funding for a carers' support project, but such effectiveness is not the whole of the story (Henwood and Waddington, 2002). For some clients, the process – the human value of being there and appearing interested and supportive – is as important as a tangible output, particularly for clients with chronic needs whose circumstances are not easily changed (Sainsbury, 1975). Cheetham et al. (1992) also urge us to differentiate effectiveness from evaluation. Evaluation judges the intrinsic worth of an activity, rather than its outcome. This acknowledges that social work can be about caring, and not necessarily about practical change. This may be contrasted with the medical model which is concerned with treatment and cure. With this in mind, we can evaluate the contribution of different sorts of service.

Evaluating day services

Day services have always played an important role in maintaining people in the community, but the advent of community care, with its emphasis on individual care planning, contracting and interagency cooperation, provides an opportunity for a reappraisal of why such services exist, for whom and with what effect. The traditional way of providing day services has been through the use of dedicated 'centres'. There are a number of different models of day centre functioning, but even though objectives may be stated in terms of only one or two models, the competing needs of users and service systems almost invariably result in centres attempting to fulfil a number of different functions, ranging from work experience to further education, to social care (Seed, 1988).

Drop-in centres have less of a care element, but may provide advice and assistance, for example about welfare benefits and other services, as well as offering a place to meet. They operate on an 'open-door' basis, but may have a core membership. Local authorities may provide funding through grant aid or contract. Membership organisations for people with mental health problems, such as Rethink, operate drop-in centres that may employ professional staff but which are managed by service users. They may give advice on dealing with other aspects of the formal psychiatric system as well as providing support and social contact. Membership is fluid and written records may not be kept.

Influence of community care on day services

Community care's commitment to wider user choice should mean the greater development of more individual programmes of care, rather than fitting people into existing resources. In order to achieve this, attention needs to be paid to the appropriateness of services; in particular, services for people from ethnic minorities are underdeveloped (SSI, 1998) and those with the most complex degree of disability are often offered the least amount of service (Mencap, 1995). To facilitate choice, care managers will also need to have access to spot contracts to buy in from a range of resources. Paradoxically, local authority funding has a tendency to push the independent sector into catering for those with higher levels of need, rather than those in the middle range. This in turn may lead to the preferred model being 'care' rather than self-development through social and leisure pursuits.

In its report on daycare services for people with mental illness, the Social Work Services Inspectorate for Scotland found that just referring someone to a service is not sufficient; to ensure that people with the greatest needs are included, a well-planned introduction and follow-up home visits are essential to secure attendance. In practice, individual follow-up at times of crisis is sometimes difficult to provide, being partly attributable to a high degree of reliance on voluntary or sessional workers. The absence of a continuing care management role is particularly problematic for the functions of monitoring and review, where day services often fulfil the role of care coordinator (under the CPA) by default. Also, if daycare services do not systematically draw up plans for individuals attending services, the emphasis within care management on the individualised response to needs is lost.

The future of day services

Clark (2001, p. 12) sees the concept of day services as obsolescent; daytime support is not necessarily or best provided within the often institutional structure of centres:

Day care can and should act as a point of access or gateway to other services needed by users. Equally, relying on traditional categories such as 'old people' or 'people with mental health problems' may narrow thinking unnecessarily and unhelpfully.

The paucity of investment in day services is apparent; day services consume only 3.4 per cent of the total expenditure on long-term care services (Royal Commission on Long Term Care, 1999). In the absence of a systematic base of research and evaluation, Clark (2001) suggests that daycare needs to be:

- more flexible in time
- more flexible in place
- more responsive to individuals' requirements
- more adaptable to variable and complex needs
- culturally and ethnically sensitive
- inclusive of disadvantaged groups
- supportive of wider social integration.

In addition, he sees carers as needing more support from day services which should be aiming not just to provide them with respite, but to involve them in short- and long-term planning. Fragmentation of services may, however, affect the usefulness of day services as sources of support to carers, if a consistent and supportive relationship cannot be built up.

Evaluating home support services

Developing the role of home support services is absolutely fundamental to community care. Providing support for people to remain living in their own homes is the first service option presented in *Community Care in the Next Decade and Beyond: Policy Guidance* (DoH, 1990a). 'Home support services' is the generic term used by the SSI (1995) to describe a range of tasks which may also be subsumed under the title of 'domiciliary or home care'. These are:

- personal assistance with daily living activities
- domestic help with household tasks
- social and emotional support.

The attributes of such services are that they should be sufficient, reliable, coordinated, flexible and affordable and based on values which are shared between users and providers of services. These values are autonomy, respect, participation, knowledge, fulfilment, privacy and equality (SSI, 1995).

The definition of home support services to include personal, domestic and emotional support is highly ambitious, given the history of service development in domiciliary care. It was an earlier SSI report (1987) which encouraged local authorities to move from providing a home help (cleaning) service towards providing a home care (personal care) service, with the result that nowadays a domestic cleaning service, although favoured by service users and arguably a statutory requirement under the Chronically Sick and Disabled Persons Act 1970, is rarely available from the public sector to people who do not also have personal care needs (RADAR, 1992; Age Concern, 1994). The provision of 'social and emotional support' (service component 3) is rarely specifically provided for in care plans, given the rationing of home care tasks by time and function. The development of close, confiding relationships between home care staff and service users is also threatened by frequent staff changes and discontinuities in services. The SSI (1995) report recognises that this is an aspect of the service that has drawn critical comment from the local government ombudsman. More fundamentally, consideration must be given to the disempowering nature of domiciliary care for people, particularly older women. The feelings of those who once took pride in doing tasks for themselves need to be sensitively addressed. There is evidence of a higher incidence of depression amongst users of domiciliary services than amongst the general population (Robertson, 1995).

Home support services as a concept is capable of wider interpretation than traditional home help or home care services. There is a perceived large unmet need for low-level practical support to enable older people in particular to remain at home in their own communities. Raynes et al. (2001) explored older people's own ideas of what a quality home care service should look like; the provision of companionship, safe transport and better healthcare were seen as important factors affecting people's attitudes to living comfortably at home. Help with basic housework, a flexible attitude to tasks and help to 'get away from the four walls' were seen as important attributes. On a personal level, continuity of carers and advance notice of changes was seen as contributing to security and confidence.

Private providers of domiciliary care, after a fairly slow start, accounted for about 23 per cent of the market by 1993 (Kestenbaum, 1993). Their growth was promoted by the requirement that local authorities spend 85 per cent of the transfer element of their special transitional grant money (from former social security funding) in the independent sector. By 2002, 64 per cent of the total contact hours of home care were provided by the independent sector (DoH, 2002f). As part of the Outcomes of Social Care for Adults project, Patmore (2001) investigated aspects of service organisation, resources and commissioning arrangements which make a home care service able to respond to older people's individual values, preferences and requests within the guidance in FACS. Although Burgner (1996) recommended the registration and inspection of domiciliary care agencies, their position was unregulated until the coming into force of the Care Standards Act 2000. All such agencies are now required to register with the CSCI, according to National Minimum Standards and Regulations. These new National Minimum Standards will require a greater investment in training by domiciliary care agencies. Compliance will be monitored through contract specifications and the monitoring and review process.

Evaluating residential care

Although deinstitutionalisation was a motivation in promoting care in the community, the peculiar status of residential care remains. Residential care may either be considered as 'an alternative to community care' (Alaszewski and Wun,

1994) or part of it (Peace et al., 1997). It is not living at home, but it is part of care in the community. Residential care covers a wide spectrum, from large residential homes of 35-plus residents to small fully staffed group homes in ordinary residential locations. Although much of the literature on residential care is concerned with older people, only 5 per cent of the population over 65 lives in residential care. Residential care, widely defined, is still significant for people with learning disabilities; 35 per cent of people with learning disabilities under the age of 65 live in residential care (SSI, 1997). In addition to these figures, there are more people passing through residential care on a short-term basis. Some of these will join mainstream residential care, whilst others will be accommodated in specialist resources.

It is important, however, to be clear about the purpose of any such service and the means chosen to achieve it, before identifying appropriate indicators by which to judge its performance (Stalker, 1996). Different criteria, for example, would be used to evaluate a short-term care break intended to be a holiday from those intended for medical assessment. The use of language again is significant – whether 'respite care', 'shared care', 'breaks and opportunities' or 'community links' – as each of these terms connotes a different balance between care and dependency and independence and opportunity.

Within residential care services, aspects of quality assurance and quality control have been given greater prominence than monitoring and review functions (see Chapter 6). This is due to the legal requirement of registration and inspection originally contained in the Residential Homes Act 1984, now the Care Standards Act 2000. However, for the resident, issues of monitoring and review may have greater importance because they are the individualised expressions of quality and a means of evaluating whether the resource provided actually meets the needs of the service user as an individual. The common practice of holding reviews as early as four weeks after admission to residential care to confirm permanency may not in all cases give residents or their families time to make an informed choice.

From its inception, it was acknowledged that community care could not replace residential provision for the most vulnerable people and the White Paper (DoH, 1989) said as much. This is despite the assertion of Wagner (1988) that people should not have to change the place in which they live in order to receive the care that they need. It remains true, however, that the best institutions are those that have permeable boundaries and strong links with the communities within which they are located (Jack, 1998). The number of supported residents in residential and nursing homes has increased from a baseline of 100,000 in 1993 to 284,100 in 2003, although this now includes former preserved rights residents who had been supported through the social security system as they were in residential care prior to 1993. Seventy-eight per cent of all supported residents are aged 65 or over; demographic pressures have therefore meant that the residential care sector remains an important part of publicly funded support for vulnerable, particularly older, adults. The greatest change over time has been in the provision of local authority residential care; only 12 per cent of residents financially supported by the local authority are in fact in local authority staffed homes. The idea of residential care as part of a continuum of housing provision in the community is further explored in Chapter 11.

What works

The PSSRUs at the Universities of Kent, York and Manchester are undertaking a number of research programmes evaluating the process and outcomes of community care (PSSRU Bulletin, 2003, at www.pssru.ac.uk). As the policy agenda has evolved over the last five years, the research programmes have been adjusted to incorporate the partnership agenda and associated moves towards the greater integration of health and social care. Outcomes from the Evaluating Community Care for Older People Project (PSSRU Bulletin, 2003) suggest that the targeting of community care services can reduce the probability of admission to hospital by over 20 per cent, and the following relationships were found:

- Home care reduces hospital admissions particularly for stroke victims and users with significant problems in undertaking activities of daily living
- Day services are most effective for users living alone
- Respite care reduces the probability of admission for older people who had come into contact with social services following an inpatient care episode
- Community nursing inputs reduce admissions for users with informal care.

In anticipation of the single assessment process for older people, the PSSRU at the University of Manchester (www.pssru.ac.uk) has undertaken a randomised control trial which found that compared to a standard social services assessment, a specialist healthcare assessment was particularly successful in detecting cognitive impairment and depression. What is acknowledged as missing is an effective tool for canvassing the views of older people concerning their satisfaction with services (Bauld et al., 2000). The National Institute for Social Work (NISW) has looked at the effectiveness of services for people with dementia in terms of supporting them successfully in the community and has reported service user and carer opinions (Moriarty and Webb, 2000). The research found that social workers used services such as domiciliary care, daycare and respite care as a hierarchy of interventions. Although the degree of cognitive impairment was the most significant indicator of future admission to residential care, daycare in particular was effective in delaying that admission. Respite care also enabled carers to maintain their support for longer and there was no evidence in this study that the use of respite care was more likely to precipitate people into full-time care by closing up their social space in the community.

Concluding comments

The proceduralisation of social work practice has been a theme of this chapter. Recent research has confirmed earlier findings that greater emphasis is placed on assessment than monitoring and review within the process of care management. Time spent on face-to-face contact with service users and carers is subordinated to indirect work in liaising with other agencies and service providers. The provision of services has been shown to be sensitive to changes in philosophy and demand. Although this type of infrastructure work in developing services is valuable and appropriate to working with communities, there are some concerns that 'good' practice has been subordinated to 'accountable' practice in the process of review. Service users, providers and commissioners all have an interest in the quality of services. Both internal and external mechanisms exist for assuring quality and these are examined in Chapter 6. A fundamental question is: whose definition of quality will prevail, and what is the proper interpretation of good professional practice?

PAUSE AND REFLECT

Construct a role play of a review of services for a person with complex needs who may be in receipt of a range of community care services. Take the role of chair of the review. Who should be invited to the review? How can you ensure that all views are represented in the discussion? Can you construct an agenda which will look at needs holistically?

CASE STUDY

Monitoring and review

Gary Lewis is 19 years old and has just begun a computer course at his local college of further education. Gary has cystic fibrosis and is a wheelchair user. He currently lives with his parents who assist with personal care and physiotherapy. The need for such assistance fluctuates from week to week; sometimes limited help is needed, at other times a lot of assistance is required. Gary is talking about leaving home to live with his friend Jack, who he has met at college. Jack would not, however, be able to provide the kind of assistance that Gary's parents now provide. Gary approaches a local independent living group for assistance.

Assuming that Gary could be supported in moving in with Jack, what arrangements would need to be put in place for the adequacy of his personal assistance to be monitored and reviewed?

FURTHER READING

Clark, C. (2001) *Adult Day Services and Social Inclusion*. London: Jessica Kingsley.
Little has been written about the function and structure of day services for adults. This book explores the movement away from institutional day centre provision to day services as a resource within long-term care services to support service users and carers.

Cooper, J. (2002) *The Care Homes Legal Handbook*. London: Jessica Kingsley.
An introduction to the new regulatory framework for care homes introduced by the Care Standards Act 2000. Includes discussion of the impact of the Human Rights Act, complaints procedures and the care homes tribunal, and staff employment and training issues.

Stalker, K. (ed.) (1996) *Developments in Short-term Care: Breaks and Opportunities*. London: Jessica Kingsley.
Explores the provision of short-term care for different user groups and looks at the different ways in which short breaks may be used and evaluated.

CHAPTER 6

Quality Assurance and Quality Control

Introduction

This chapter explores the ways in which the decisions of public authorities may be challenged. Forms of redress that people might seek range from a simple apology to the use of a complaints procedure or legal action. It also explores good administrative practice through the examination of some decisions of the local government ombudsman and also examines the impact of the Human Rights Act 1998 on the way in which services are provided. Accountability to service users requires their definition of quality to contribute to standards for the services provided and the social work practice which supports them.

KEY ROLE 5

Manage and be accountable, with supervision and support, for your own social work practice within your organisation

---

Ways of defining quality

Quality assurance and quality control are important means by which standards of service are set and maintained. 'Quality assurance' is the term used to refer to those processes which aim to ensure that concern for quality is designed and built into services. 'Quality control' refers to processes of verification or challenge and will include systematic monitoring, audit and inspection, designed to establish whether standards are being achieved. 'Total quality management' describes an approach to quality assurance which stresses the importance of creating a culture in which concern for quality is an integral part of service delivery (DoH, 1992).

This procedural approach to quality assurance does not answer the question of who defines what quality is in any particular service. Is it to be the service user, the commissioner of that service (the local authority), or the provider of this service? If the answer is 'a combination of all three', then whose voice is the most powerful, particularly where consumer choice is limited through both rationing processes and the absence of providers? As issues of quality are explored, it may be helpful to keep in mind Pfeffer and Coote's (1991) perspectives on 'what is quality?' Is it:

- the achievement of standards set by experts?
- a reflection of prestige or positional advantage?
- a managerial wish to achieve excellence – as measured by user satisfaction?
- empowerment of the service user?

This is a theme which will be returned to throughout this chapter. Quality assurance and quality control take place within a framework of rights, duties and remedies, which are all interlinked. However, the assertion of a right in the abstract is of little value if there is no remedy for enforcing that right (if the local authority, for example, does not provide the service needed). The development of accessible and effective remedies is therefore crucial not only to enforce rights in individual cases, but also authoritatively to interpret and develop the law.

Quality assurance in these circumstances means adherence to the principles of good administration: openness, fairness and accountability. Although these are procedural rather than substantive rights, they are not inconsiderable, as will be discussed below.

Trends within quality assurance and quality control

Following *Modernising Social Services* (DoH, 1998a), the emphasis has shifted in favour of greater formal regulation and an acknowledgement that users and carers have an essential voice in the setting of quality standards at the policy level and their monitoring in practice. The Care Standards Act 2000 created an entirely new arm's-length body, the National Care Standards Commission (now the Commission for Social Care Inspection – CSCI), to regulate services both in the independent and public sector (see www.csci.org.uk). Best value requirements and performance indicators also set national standards against which local performance is measured. The term 'quality', however, is misused if it is seen only as an operational term to describe a particular set of institutionalised review activities. As the DoH report *Committed to Quality* (1992) itself found, the creation of inspectorate or review processes may assist in that process but their creation does not ensure quality; it simply ensures that systems exist to measure it (DoH, 1992, para. 2.15).

Measures of outcome may be different for each of the stakeholders, for example a value for money service that conforms to legal requirements may do nothing to improve the subjective experience of the service user. Evaluation of a service is particularly problematic when that service is personal care (Hughes, 1995), given the constraints on users and carers expressing dissatisfaction with a service on which they rely.

An outcomes approach to quality

The *Outcomes of Social Care for Adults* (OSCA) programme (Henwood and Waddington, 2002) was the first sustained exploration of social care outcomes for adults since 1993 and the introduction of community care. The change of emphasis since 1993 is described in terms of two stages: the first stage being the monitoring of progress made in changing systems and the second the collecting of evidence of the difference such changes have made to the lives of service users. 'Process outcomes', examining the impact of service changes on people's experience of systems, for example changes to carers assessments, may nevertheless have a potent influence on final outcomes for users and carers. Understanding and defining outcomes is a contested enterprise: the outcomes of social care are multidimensional and different stakeholders have differing perspectives. Henwood and Waddington (2002) also identify polarities in defining outcomes between:

- intermediate   and   final
- short term   and   long term
- subjective   and   objective
- individual   and   aggregated.

The National Occupational Standards for Social Work (TOPSS, 2002) focus not on user outcomes, but on process outcomes and key roles relevant to that process. They focus on the competence of the worker to perform the range of tasks within the care management process. Other difficulties are that there may be no baseline from which change can clearly be measured, and the outcome achieved, or intended, may not be change so much as maintenance; it is also rarely possible to make comparisons with similar non-intervention control groups when equally vulnerable people are considered. Desired outcomes have also evolved from a general concern with maintaining people in the community to a focus on promoting independence, maximising individual capacity and achieving rehabilitation objectives (Henwood and Waddington, 2002, p. i).

Is this formal identification of concern with outcomes reflected in the actual experiences of service users? Researching the experiences of disabled service users, Priestley (2003) notes high levels of satisfaction with self-managed support where individual choice and control are prioritised, contrasting this with the lack of flexibility shown by both statutory and independent agencies, and the 'burden of gratitude' which may be attached to support from friends and family. Recognising that measuring quality may variously be defined in terms of either self-reported well-being, tangible outcomes, change over time, or 'active citizenship', Priestley is sceptical about the motives behind formal systems' espousal of quality of life measures. As he states (2003, p. 185):

> The increasing attention on quality of life issues within commissioning authorities has been driven not so much by concern for the citizenship of disabled people as by the bureaucratic imperatives to ration scarce resources.

Measuring quality

Research by Vernon and Qureshi (2000), based on focus groups of disabled people, produced similar findings. Service users themselves defined independent living in terms of access to and control of services enabling individuals to pursue their own lifestyle, whilst professionals prioritised personal care over social support, and defined independence as self-sufficiency. Process outcomes were also seen by users as important aspects of empowerment and user control. Important issues here were the provision of sufficient information to support choice, waiting times, value for money and the competence of staff. Wilson and Beresford (2002) take the debate on definitions of quality into the arena of anti-oppressive practice, noting that recipients of social work services have been minimally involved in discussions and initiatives associated with the development of anti-oppressive practice and the question of who is qualified or authorised to determine what counts as anti-oppressive. The different perspectives inevitably come into conflict when the disabled people's movement is increasingly focusing on rights and citizenship and organisational discourses are still focused on defining and differentiating welfare needs.

The process of care planning also involves issues of quality in relation to contract compliance (Hughes, 1995). Research amongst consumers has shown a real concern for quality, particularly as regards domiciliary care, where until recently there was no legislative framework for registration and standard-setting (Robertson, 1995; Harding and Beresford, 1996). But whether or not refusing to accept a less than appropriate standard of care is a realistic prospect depends on the availability of alternatives, which may in turn be limited by the local authority's choice of approved providers in the contracting system (Kestenbaum, 1993).

Quality mechanisms in residential care

Local authority residential care has historically been less closely regulated than the independent sector. Reliance has been placed largely on the demands of professionalism and political accountability. The Care Standards Act 2000 introduces a new category of 'care home' and covers both the local authority and independent sector equally. Increasingly, there is a diversity of standards to be attained beyond the registration baseline – age, sex, number of residents, category of persons accommodated. For example, the current National Minimum Standards and Care Home Regulations for Adults 18–65 run to 138 pages, and include supplementary standards for young people aged 16 and 17 (DoH, 2003). They cover:

- Choice of home (including needs assessments and introductory visits)
- Individual needs and choices (including service user plans, decision-making and confidentiality)
- Lifestyle (including personal development, leisure and relationships)
- Personal and healthcare support
- Concerns, complaints and protection
- The environment
- Staffing
- Conduct and management of the home (including record-keeping and safe working practices).

The standards also include outcome measures. For example, the outcome measure for planned admissions is that each service user has an individual written contract or statement of terms and conditions within the home. Local authorities may also introduce additional specification standards in their contracts with the private sector. Market forces therefore will be a potent factor in honing and enhancing standards in each sector of care. Beyond this there exists the Care Standards Tribunal which hears appeals against the refusal or cancellation of registration. There is also an emergency procedure (Care Standards Act 2000, s.14) whereby the CSCI can apply for an order from a magistrates' court for the immediate cancellation of registration. The registration and inspection of residential care faces problems common to all regulatory systems: policing v. consultancy, rules v. discretion, stringency v. accommodation (Day et al., 1996). Paradoxically, some aspects of the system may be intended to pose difficulties:

> registration is deliberately designed as an obstacle course (a sort of initiation ceremony) that forces prospective home owners to demonstrate that they are 'fit persons', that their plans meet local guidelines and that they know what is expected of them. (Day et al., 1996)

User outcomes

More recently, user outcomes have been incorporated into inspection practice. The enhanced role of the CSCI, following the amalgamation of the National Care Standards Commission with the Social Services Inspectorate and the SSI/Audit Commission Joint Review Team, includes the assessment of value for money of council social services and the publication of star ratings. Since the same service can assist different people in different ways, it will be important to evaluate service outcomes for individuals, as well as research the performance of a service as a whole. This means that the social worker's task of providing information by which the authority can show that it has met performance indicators must be set alongside the professional need for reflective practice as a source of evaluation and learning (Nocon and Qureshi, 1996, p. 21). Personalising outcomes in this way is in turn dependent on a needs-led rather than resource-led approach to assessment at the beginning of the care management process. If process involves giving time to the service user, empathising and ensuring choice and accessibility in services, it is likely to secure a good outcome.

Here, as elsewhere, a distinction exists between exit and voice models of empowerment (Hirschman, 1970; Bewley and Glendinning, 1994). Within the market model, users are expected to react to agencies' agendas, rather than propose the issues they themselves see as most important. 'Voice' means being involved in making decisions and potentially also evaluating the outcome of those decisions in a way which leads to positive change. 'Exit' is based on free-market principles, whereby service users are free to go elsewhere if services do not meet their needs. Exit may also be linked to complaints procedures as part of quality control, if dissatisfaction with services is to be highlighted. The difficulty is that very often the service user is in no position to exit the system on which his or her safety or well-being depends. The following discussion on remedies in community care focuses on this notion of quality control in terms of remedies

Remedies in community care

There is an increasing awareness, from a consumer perspective, that the decisions of local authorities are challengeable in a number of ways (see McDonald, 1997). This includes a willingness to take legal action to support claims to legal rights. The existence of effective remedies is a necessary fourth element in the paradigm of rights, powers, duties and remedies, depending on whether what is sought is an apology, compensation or a changed decision (Payne, 1995).

Complaints procedures

Section 50 of the NHSCCA 1990 inserted a new section 7B into the Local Authority Social Services Act 1970, requiring local authorities to set up representations and complaints procedures to operate in respect of matters arising after 1 April, 1991. There is evidence, however, that wide variations exist in interpretation and process throughout the country (SSI, 1993; Connolly, 1996).

Under this procedure, complaints must be made within a time limit of six months by and in respect of a 'qualifying individual'. According to the Local Authority Social Services Act, s.7B(2), a person is a qualifying individual if:

- a local authority has a power or duty to provide, or to secure the provision of, a social service for him or her
- his or her need or possible need for such a service has (by whatever means) come to the attention of the local authority.

Local authorities may, at their discretion, deal with representations or complaints outside these categories. A wide variety of issues may be addressed:

> Complaints can result from an unresolved problem or from a measure of dissatisfaction or disquiet about the organisation, about the quality and appropriateness of services, or about their delivery or non-delivery. (DoH, 1990a, para. 6.7)

Complaints procedures should be kept separate from grievance procedures and disciplinary procedures which concern internal staffing matters.

The procedures themselves are in three stages: an informal stage, a formal stage and a review panel stage. If the matter cannot be resolved to the satisfaction of the complainant after informal discussion, he or she should be invited to submit a written representation and should be given assistance and guidance in the use of the formal procedure, or advice on where she or he can obtain such assistance. A major difficulty in practice is getting systems to recognise that an expression of dissatisfaction is in fact a complaint. A formal written complaint becomes a 'registered' complaint to which the authority should respond within 28 days. Alternatively, the local authority should explain why a response within that time is not possible and advise the complainant when he or she can expect a response, which in any case should be given within three months. Complaints concerning voluntary and private sector provision contracted for through the local authority should, wherever possible, be handled at the informal stage by the service provider (DoH, 1990a, para. 31). Complainants who are dissatisfied with the response they receive, or who do not wish to complain to the service provider, may choose to refer the matter to the local authority; complaints received by this route should be treated as registered complaints.

If the complainant informs the authority in writing within 28 days of notification of the outcome of the formal stage that he or she is still dissatisfied and wishes the matter to be referred to a panel for review, the local authority is required to convene a panel to meet within 28 days of the request. The review panel should be made up of three people, one of whom should be independent of the local authority. Complaints procedures under section 26(3) of the Children Act 1989 differ in that they require an independent element at the second stage as well. Ten days notice should be given, during which written submissions may be made. There is a right to an oral hearing, and a right to be accompanied by or represented by some other person at the hearing, although legal representation is excluded. The panel's decision takes the form of a recommendation to the director of social services, and although the recommendation is not binding, its persuasive value is considerable. The proper operation of local authority complaints procedures also comes within the jurisdiction of the ombudsman, whose concern is with due process issues, and for whom the operation of complaints procedures has raised issues of fairness and undue delay.

The CSCI plans to assume responsibility for the review of complaints about local authority SSDs under the Health and Social Care (Community Standards) Act 2003. The intention is to harmonise complaints for adults and children. Key areas for improvement were identified in a Department of Health consultation (2000d) as:

- Time limits for eligibility to make a complaint
- Timescales for investigation
- Timescales for local resolution
- The investigative role of the independent person
- The right to advocacy
- 'Freezing' decisions during the complaints process
- Implementing decisions
- Boundaries between different complaints procedures.

Complaints procedures within the NHS are subject to an informal stage of local resolution followed by a request to a complaints convenor for an independent review on a discretionary basis. A national evaluation of the NHS complaints procedure highlighted widespread dissatisfaction with the level of independence and lengthy nature of the procedure for independent review (DoH, 2001g). The Health and Social Care (Community Standards) Act 2003 has given the CHAI the duty of undertaking reviews of complaints which are outstanding after local resolution procedures have been exhausted. The complainant will have a further right to a hearing by a panel of three independent lay people. Where complaints involve different aspects of care such as a PCT, NHS trust or ambulance trust, the CHAI will be able to look at the whole of the patient's experience. Information from complaints will be used to improve services locally. Complainants will also to be able to pursue a complaint at the same time as taking legal action.

Ombudsmen

The idea of using ombudsmen to investigate complaints of maladministration in public service comes from Scandinavia and was first introduced into England and Wales in 1967. The system now covers both central and local government as well as the NHS; it has also extended into the commercial field of finance. The system is a useful one where a complaint is about procedures or confusion and delay rather than the quality of a decision already made. Although complaints are individualised, very often patterns can be discerned, and the reports of ombudsmen are a useful political tool to highlight difficulties in the implementation of policy.

The local government ombudsman (or, formally, the Commissioner for Local Administration) may investigate allegations of injustice caused by maladministration in the performance of its functions by a local authority. Maladministration is generally taken to mean those matters contained in the so-called Crossman catalogue (H.C. Deb., col. 51, 18 October 1966): 'Bias, neglect, inattention, delay, incompetence, ineptitude, arbitrariness and the like.' The function of the ombudsman is thus to uphold principles of good administration, not to question the merits of a decision – for that the complaints procedure should be used. Referrals must be made within 12 months and alternative rights and remedies must already have been exhausted, unless the ombudsman feels it is not reasonable to expect the complainant to use these rights. The complainant will usually apply in person, but where he or she is unable to do so, 'some body or individual suitable to represent him' may apply on his behalf (Local Government Act, 1974 s.27(2)). An attempt is usually made to achieve a settlement without a formal investigation and only 5 per cent of complaints actually result in a final report. A copy of the final report will be sent to all the parties, and if the local authority does not act upon his recommendation, the ombudsman may publish a further report leading to a statement in an agreed form which must be published in the local press.

The ombudsman has been quite stringent in his criticism of local authorities for their failure to implement good practice. Complaints of delay in responding to requests for assessment or the delivery of services are frequently made and, on the whole, priority criteria for assessment have not protected local authorities from criticism. In one of a series of complaints against Liverpool City Council alleging delays in assessment and the provision of occupational therapy services, the ombudsman saw fit to lay down maximum time limits of two months for urgent cases and six months for non-urgent cases; although these sound generous, they are in fact quite modest deadlines for some authorities who have a shortage of qualified staff and resources. A recent innovation has been for the ombudsman in some cases to require local authorities to report back to him in three months' time on progress made in reforming systems. The ombudsman may recommend that small amounts of compensation are awarded to those who suffer injustice as a consequence of maladministration.

The parliamentary ombudsman investigates complaints against government departments and certain non-departmental public bodies. MPs are used as the filter to refer complaints on to the ombudsman. Investigations may involve the reading of government files and papers, and the consideration of oral evidence, and are held in private. Compensation may be paid on an ex gratia basis, but again the investigation is into maladministration and not into the merits of a decision.

Although the power of the ombudsman is formally limited to publicising shortcomings in services in individual cases, the influence of the ombudsman's reports can extend far beyond this, into the field of policy. This is particularly true of the health service ombudsman whose special investigations into the continuing care needs of patients transferred to nursing home care from the NHS have led to a review of policy on continuing care and subsequent guidance from the Department of Health (see Chapter 10).

Default powers

In the field of public law, if a local authority fails to carry out any of its statutory duties, the secretary of state can declare the authority to be in default, issue directions to ensure that the duties specified are complied with and, if necessary, enforce those directions in the High Court. The process is a discretionary one, and there is no recorded instance of the power having been used, although the secretary of state may enter into correspondence with local authorities against which complaints have been made. Placing authorities under 'special measures' when performance indicators have not been met is the administrative equivalent of default powers, and is used when there is concern about quality.

Legal actions

Using the authority of the courts to enforce rights to service, or procedural rights to fair assessment and service allocation, is likely to become an important avenue of complaint. The actions of local authorities can be challenged before the courts in private and public law. *Private law actions* are concerned with individual rights and their objective is the clarification and enforcement of duties owed to individuals, not the public at large. Those who bring private law actions seek individual remedies such as injunctions and damages. Such actions are based on ordinary principles of contract and tort. *Public law actions* are often brought as test cases in order to clarify the law for the benefit of others as well. The remedies sought will emphasise the public rather than the private interest in having decisions properly made, and may be concerned more with procedural irregularities than substantive issues; damages by way of compensation will be available only in a minority of cases.

Private law rights

Despite the rhetoric of community care in claiming to incorporate users' rights into the provision of services, legal remedies for the enforcement of such rights are not much in evidence. The concept of a legal contract as a 'bargain' freely entered into by parties will in most cases not fit the reality of block service agreements whose terms are not variable in individual cases. Harden (1992), discussing NHS contracts, makes the same point; the law does not provide a coherent framework for consumers' rights or for the separation of interests where public bodies provide or contract for services.

Some claims which can be brought in contract may also be brought in the tort of negligence, the basis of which is breach of a duty of care owed to another as a consequence of which that other person suffers damage which is foreseeable. An example might be of a care home which fails to provide an adequate number of trained staff. If, as a consequence of lack of oversight, a resident should fall and injure him or herself, it is likely that he/she would have a cause of action in negligence against the owner of the home. That owner could, of course, be the local authority, in which case the local authority would be liable. But what if the home was providing a placement under a contractual arrangement with the local authority? The local authority will not be liable unless it was itself negligent. It may have been negligent, for example, in continuing to make placements there when alerted by complaints that staffing was inadequate.

A further cause of action may exist not in negligence but in an action for breach of statutory duty. For there to be liability to individuals, the test is whether or not the statute intended to give them this benefit. This is not often found to be the case; the usual interpretation is that statutory duties are owed only to the public at large. An example is the duty placed upon the secretary of state for health by section 1 of the National Health Service Act 1977 to provide a comprehensive health service – a provision which has been unsuccessfully challenged by patients unhappy at the curtailing of NHS facilities. Such a duty is sometimes described as a target duty operating on the political rather than the legal plane (Cragg, 1996). However, some specific duties may be owed to individuals so as to found an action for breach of statutory duty. An example of a duty owed in private law is the duty in section 2 of the Chronically Sick and Disabled Persons Act 1970 to make arrangements to meet the assessed needs of persons with a disability. This private law right to sue the local authority if services are not forthcoming survives the decision of the House of Lords in the Gloucestershire case (discussed in Chapter 2), provided the local authority's eligibility criteria have been met.

Public law rights

Applications for judicial review are the primary legal means of enforcing public law duties. Application is to the administrative court. The process is both complex and costly and may be undertaken only by persons with a sufficient interest in the matter in dispute. However, judicial review is being used increasingly on a test case basis to clarify the statutory responsibilities of public bodies such as local authorities, health authorities, government departments and prison boards of visitors. The Child Poverty Action Group, RADAR and Help the Aged have brought actions in this way.

It is the legality of an action – whether that action is assessing resources for residential care, or limiting services by way of eligibility criteria – rather than the merits of a decision which is challenged in this way. Judicial review is also used to challenge decisions taken without due process, with inadequate consultation or in contradiction of already publicised criteria. Decisions to close homes for older people have been successfully challenged for inadequate consultation with resident groups. Now that local authorities are required to be explicit about assessment procedures and service availability in accordance with the principles of open government, judicial review might usefully be considered to hold such authorities to account for their actions.

Impact of the Human Rights Act 1998

The Human Rights Act 1998 came into force in October 2000. Effectively, it incorporates the majority of the provisions of the 1951 European Convention on Human Rights into English law, by requiring the courts to interpret national legislation to be compatible with the rights given in the Convention, wherever possible. This means that the Convention rights can have a direct effect in the UK without individuals needing to access the European Court of Human Rights in Strasbourg for their enforcement against the state in individual cases. The impact of the Human Rights Act is potentially profound, as all new legislation contains a preamble saying that it is believed to be compatible with the Convention; furthermore, the higher courts have the power to declare both Acts of Parliament and regulations made under them 'incompatible', indicating to Parliament a need for a change in the law. The rights contained in the European Convention are primarily individual civil and political rights, rather than collective economic and social rights (McDonald, 2001).

However, since it is unlawful for public authorities to act in contravention of these rights, the Human Rights Act effectively gives a new ground of challenge to the use of powers by any arm of the state. Although some rights, such as the right to protection from torture and inhuman and degrading treatment (Article 3), are absolute, some rights are limited, for example Article 5, the right to liberty, contains within it exceptions to this right such as the power of arrest or detention for psychiatric treatment. Given the complexity of civil society and the need to balance rights and responsibilities, some rights are qualified rights. Examples are the right to respect for private and family life (Article 8) and the right to freedom of expression (Article 10). States may thus lawfully interfere in family life, for example by taking children into care, or may limit freedom of expression through the law of defamation. Although these rights are qualified, there are safeguards; interference with them is permissible only if what is done:

- has its basis in law
- is necessary in a democratic society, which means it must
  - ❏ fulfil a pressing social need
  - ❏ pursue a legitimate aim
  - ❏ be proportionate to the aims being pursued.

In addition, in international law, states are given a 'margin of appreciation' in interpreting the Convention in accordance with their own cultural traditions and social policy.

The European Convention imposes positive duties to protect vulnerable individuals, and the obligation to have procedures to deal with abuse has led to the development of law and policy in this area in the UK (see Chapter 4). In some circumstances, the state's duty to protect may extend to the provision of resources. So, in the case of *Bernard* v. *Enfield LBC* (McDonald, 2004), a disabled mother of six children successfully argued that the failure of the local authority to provide her with suitable living accommodation had breached Article 8 – the right of her and her husband to family life. The conditions in which she was living, in an unadapted property where she was unable to access basic facilities, failed only by a narrow margin also to reach the threshold of degrading treatment set by Article 3. The importance to public authorities of ensuring that they conform to the Human Rights Act is apparent. This obligation will sit alongside responsibilities to conform to anti-discriminatory legislation on race, gender, sexual orientation and belief, both in the development of policy and the implementation of decisions. It is also the responsibility of each individual social worker not only to be familiar with the requirements of the Human Rights Act, but also to be proactive in supporting a positive attitude to human rights issues (McDonald, 2001).

The impact of the Human Rights Act must not, however, be exaggerated. A study by the Audit Commission in 2004 found that although awareness of human rights issues had increased, 58 per cent of public authorities surveyed had not developed a strategy for human rights, and 61 per cent had not put arrangements in place to ensure that contractors were complying with the Act. This is of concern, given the limiting effect of the ruling in the Leonard Cheshire Homes case (McDonald, 2004) that independent care provision would normally not be considered to be a public function under the Human Rights Act so as to have its obligations imposed directly on contractors. The Audit Commission report also produces no new evidence that human rights issues are being used to develop the wider application of anti-oppressive practice (Thompson, 2003). This means that agencies or individuals within them are not extending a commitment to anti-oppressive practice into their relationships with legal advisors who can provide guidance on the interpretation of policies and decisions in line with human rights requirements.

Concluding comments

This chapter looked at ways in which the quality of service provision can be assured, through regulatory regimes and the use of complaints procedures and legal challenges. The impact of the Human Rights Act 1998 on the delivery of community care services is only just starting to be explored. It will, however, disclose basic conflicts between service users and public authorities in the definition of what constitutes an adequate service to meet fundamental rights and needs. The justification for systems of quality control in public services lies in public accountability. It empowers service users to make explicit to them the means of challenging local authority decisions. Legal actions have a particular potency because they give direct access to a major source of power in society – the courts. A major difficulty is that substantive issues (how much of what kind of service) are more difficult to challenge than procedural lapses. This is in large measure an outcome of a welfare system that is based on needs rather than rights, where the definition of quality on the whole remains in the hands of those who allocate the resources. Giving people a voice in the design of services is more potent than expecting them to exit from services they dislike, when the choice of service provider is limited and the services provided are essential to the maintenance of an adequate level of care. Social workers' changing roles within community care are examined in Chapter 7, which starts to move the discussion beyond a technical analysis of care management skills towards a focus on the interpersonal in relation to service users and carers.

PAUSE AND REFLECT

Collect information on your local authority's complaints procedure. How accessible is this information? What assistance may be given to people to use the system? What sort of redress is available – an apology, compensation, a changed decision? What sort of support might be necessary to assist service users in accessing the complaints procedure?

Obtain a copy of a inspection report on a local care home. Reports are available on the CSCI website (www.csci.org.uk). To what extent are the values of privacy, dignity, independence, choice, rights and fulfilment acknowledged in the report?

CASE STUDY

Supporting choices

Jane Morris and Stuart Smith are both in their mid-twenties and live in a care home for people with learning difficulties. They have told staff that they are a 'couple' and would like to share a room. Their intention is to get married and have their own flat. Both sets of parents object to this and want Jane and Stuart to be separated.

If you were the manager of the home, how would you deal with this situation, and what principles would guide you?

FURTHER READING

Henwood, M. and Waddington, E. (2002) *Outcomes of Social Care For Adults: Messages for Policy and Practice*. Leeds: Nuffield Institute for Health.
An overview of the DoH-sponsored OSCA programme looking at outcomes of social care services for adults. A brief overview is given of the projects within the programme which range from a study of the management and effectiveness of home care assistants to outcomes for learning disabled people in the community 12 years on. The studies update the impact of community care policy on the experiences of a range of service users and carers. The meaning and definition of 'outcomes' over time is also explored.

Shaping our Lives National User Network (2003) *Social Service Users' Own Definitions of Quality Outcomes*. York: Joseph Rowntree Foundation.
Explores the important question of who defines quality in social care, and puts forward user perspectives.

CHAPTER 7

Changing Roles

Introduction

Process issues – the ways in which social workers use interpersonal skills in their relationships with service users and carers – and the methods of intervention that they might use in dealing with complex family and social relationships are the subject matter of this chapter. Many users are clear about the personal and professional qualities that they value in workers. Multidisciplinary settings are becoming increasingly common, so working with other professionals is an important skill in current social work practice. From the outset, community care was predicated on the availability of informal support networks and carers. Conceptualising caring relationships and asking whether or not informal carers have become professionalised under the system of community care is another change of role explored in this chapter. Individual models of social work are compared with the finding, supporting and sustaining of community networks as a developmental task in which social workers under community care are properly engaged.

KEY ROLE 6

Demonstrate professional competence in social work practice

The nature of social work

The debate about how social work fits into the framework of care management is complicated by the lack of consensus on what social work really is. One view is to see social work as essentially malleable. Based as it is on a framework of statutory duties, the role and tasks of social work will change as social policy and legislation change. An alternative view of social work is that it exists not to ameliorate but to challenge the inequalities that exist in the lives of people with disabilities and older people, and in the marginalisation of offenders. Being practised in so many different settings and with diverse groups of people, 'social work actually does cover a multitude of virtues which are remarkably difficult to characterise in a conceptually tidy manner' (Davies, 1997). This chapter examines the changing role of social work under community care by looking at different models of care management and the social work skills they require, and the response of users and carers to change. The satisfactions and difficulties that social workers have encountered in the transition to community care are also described.

Jordan (1997) argues that social work is necessary to compensate vulnerable individuals when communities break up under pressure from market forces. Accordingly:

> there is a contradiction at the heart of social work, because it is spawned by market-orientated economic individualism, yet its values are those of a caring, inclusive, reciprocal community that takes collective responsibility for its members. (p. 10)

This contradiction is at the heart of community care policy itself, with its emphasis on the contract culture, rationing and regulation of scarce resources, whereas the real difficulty in people's lives may be the result of structural problems such as poverty and discrimination which market forces may help to sustain as well as create. An individualised model of social work practice needs to be set alongside models of social work which emphasise community action and collective responses to problem-solving.

Care management: can social work survive?

Different models exist for the institution of care management which distinguish to a greater or lesser extent between role and task. In a role-based system, the title of 'care manager' is simply a job description of the title holder, and carries with it no necessary presumption of the professional qualification (if any) of the person within it. This was what Griffiths (1988) envisaged when he spoke of the role of care manager in procedural terms. Care management as a task regards the process of care management as essentially one of method; a particular way of working which may be set alongside psychodynamic social work, for example, or cognitive behavioural therapy. The *Managers' Guide* (SSI/DoH, 1991a, para. 3.33) states the dichotomy nicely:

> In deciding on the appropriate model or models of care management, the authorities/ agencies will have to decide whether separate staff should be identified with specific care management responsibilities or whether staff can undertake care management as part of a wider range of responsibilities. The decision of agencies may be affected by the ease with which they are able to redeploy and recruit staff of the appropriate calibre.

The choice is thus between intensive care management or a care management approach.

Care management may also be provided on an integrated or segregated basis (para. 3.34). An integrated model, whereby all initial requests for assessment receive a care management response, is likely to overburden professionally qualified people at the apex of the social services pyramid. In its preliminary review of the operation of care management, the SSI (1993a) found such a top-heavy system to be widespread. One of its recommendations was for greater attention to be paid to the six separate levels of assessment detailed in the *Managers' Guide*, whereby only the most complex cases requiring comprehensive assessment were assigned to professionally qualified staff. Care management as a specialist service has been developed by some authorities, with the vast majority of simple or single-service referrals going to administrative or non-professionally qualified staff.

The *Managers' Guide* (SSI/DoH, 1991a) identifies five models of care management:

- the *single care manager model* – located either in separate teams or integrated in mainstream teams
- the *social entrepreneurship model* – a designated worker with devolved budgetary responsibility
- the *shared case tasks model* – tasks are shared by a combination of professionally and vocationally qualified staff
- the *administrative model* – for the coordination of inputs from other services
- the *user model* – service users act as their own care manager.

Pilling (1992) gives examples of a further model – the *multidisciplinary model* – in which a multidisciplinary team is responsible for assessment and developing a care plan for an individual, usually through the development of a keyworker system. This model has similarities to the CPA in mental health services (Chapter 12). Raiff and Shore (1993) also describe a model similar to that favoured by Huxley (1990) for use in mental health services which they call the *clinical model*, within which the provision of therapeutic help as well as services are within the domain of the care manager. Brandon and Towell (1989) describe a model of 'service brokerage' used in Canada in which the care manager acts as the agent of the service user in securing the best available package of care; as the care manager does not work for an agency, he or she has no agenda to reduce costs or ration resources. The introduction of direct payments in lieu of community care services is a partial move towards the empowerment of service users and the use of care managers as facilitators rather than as entrepreneurs of services.

Adams (1998) sees care management as changing the nature of social work practice towards proceduralism and away from theory-based and value-driven aspects of critically reflective practice. This is reflected in the competence-based approach to student assessment which emphasises outcomes and performance rather than learning. Doel and Shardlow (1998) locate the pre-eminence of accountability over professional autonomy within a system where there is increasing managerial control and a corresponding lack of support for frontline workers.

Working with other professions

Close liaison with other relevant professions – in education, housing and healthcare – has always been an important feature of social work. The advent of community care has made the need for that liaison more apparent, whilst fudging the boundaries between different professional groupings. The resulting dilemmas are neatly summarised by Øvretveit et al. (1997, p. 6) as:

> how to assess needs and work together with different professional languages, how to shift from profession-services to more interprofessional working, and how to combine team leadership with profession and agency management services.

Øvretveit et al. see the key issue as defining the 'team' and its purpose. Managers must first of all clarify whether a team exists for client coordination (referring on to each other and working in parallel) or a collective service (with shared responsibility and authority). Teams vary on a continuum, from the highly integrated, where the team's priorities are the strongest influence on the individual's work decisions, to a network team, which, although it may see the same 'type' of clients, is organised as a collection of disparate professional services, each under its own management with its own policies, priorities and procedures (Payne, 2000). The former are multidisciplinary teams, the latter are interdisciplinary, with an increasing trend towards the former in services for people with disabilities and mental health problems (DoH, 2001b). Interagency working, by contrast, is not dependent on teamwork, places less emphasis on professionals working together and concentrates rather on strategic issues and planning.

Øvretveit et al. (1997) see collaborative working as valuable for a number of reasons (the first four of which draw on work by Hallet and Birchall (1992) in childcare, but which are relevant to the objectives of community care). These are:

- Avoidance of duplication and overlap
- Reductions of gaps and discontinuities in services
- Clarification of roles and responsibilities
- The delivery of comprehensive, holistic services
- The promotion of a service driven by objectives and outcomes rather than by professional interests
- The potential for replacement of staff with closely supervised ancillaries

On the other hand, Øvretveit et al. (1997) see some disadvantages in interprofessionalism:

- A reduction of choice in the absence of a diversity of assessment and service
- The possibility of collusion against the client which is difficult to challenge
- A reluctance to pursue risky or novel solutions
- Inward-looking attitudes.

This greater emphasis on 'what gets done' rather than 'who does what' in multidisciplinarity assumes a consensus model of working based on similar values and priorities (Øvretveit et al., 1997). The major test of such cooperation is whether it can survive conflict. Dimond (1997) explores such conflicts in relation to legal rights and responsibilities. If a patient, discharged from a psychiatric hospital following involvement by a multidisciplinary team, commits a serious offence, who would be held responsible for his or her discharge? The answer would be the psychiatrist in charge of his or her case. Given this, it is not surprising that such a person would seek pre-eminence in decision-making and would suggest resources that are within his or her control. In the case of nurses working in a similar role to social workers, the nurse is bound by her professional code not to work 'beyond the limits of her competence'; thus professionally imposed limitations have the effect of restricting the transfer of skills. This has implications which favour the survival of distinct professional groupings in community care.

The status of social work within community care

Official statements on care management do little to clarify the status of social work within it. Neither the Griffiths Report (1988), the White Paper (DoH, 1989b) nor the *Policy Guidance* (DoH, 1990a) address in any detail what the role of social work is intended to be. Bamford (1990, p. 159) was prepared to contemplate that this was because:

> the new role envisaged in designing, organising and purchasing services is so fundamentally different from that currently performed that a wholly different approach is required to which social work has a contribution to make.

Post-implementation surveys of social workers within a care management system found widespread dissatisfaction with form-filling and the disempowering nature of the paperwork required to be completed (Petch, 1994; Macdonald and Myers, 1995). Lewis and Glennerster (1996) found that frontline workers were less enthusiastic than their managers about the community care changes and cited form-filling, hospital discharge procedures and the movement away from counselling as major sources of dissatisfaction. Managers themselves were showing a tendency, also observed by the SSI (1993a), to retreat from their professional role as 'supervisors' into a role as managers of budgets. The move from consensus management to general management not requiring professional qualification, which began in the NHS in the mid-1980s after the first Griffiths Report, was now being seen in SSDs (Simiç, 1996). Rummery (2002) found an emphasis on administrative models in social work with people with disabilities, with a focus on rapid throughput and extensive paperwork emphasising agency priorities. Studies of care management and older people have also described the social worker's experience in terms of greater bureaucracy, more complex administrative tasks and less opportunity for engagement with service users (Lewis and Glennester, 1996; Richards, 2000; Postle, 2001).

There are some interesting findings, however, about the importance of the coordinating role. A study by Weinberg et al. (2003) asked staff to complete a diary schedule in which job-related activities were broken down into five categories, based on previous research:

- direct contact with the older person
- contact with informal carers
- service contact related to the older person and/or carer
- procedural and organisational commitments
- travel.

The research found that:

- 18 per cent of the case managers' time was spent on direct work with the older person and 6 per cent with the carer
- 40 per cent was spent on service contact such as gathering information from other agencies, carrying out paperwork and discussions with colleagues or providers
- 25 per cent was spent on meetings and organisational commitments
- 11 per cent on travel.

The frequency of tasks confirms the prevalence of administrative and service arrangement duties and the proportion of time spent on assessment compared with monitoring and review. However, compared to pre-1993 studies, and in comparison with other professions, this piece of research did not find a significant bureaucratisation of the work. What appears to have happened is that there has been a shift within the overall broad categories such as direct work from monitoring and review to assessment. But although assessment activities took up 50 per cent of the face-to-face contact time, only 25 per cent of this time was devoted to counselling and supportive work, and a limited time was devoted to carers. Overall, the data from Weinberg et al.'s study suggests that, for the majority of their time, practitioners are engaged in a coordinating rather than a person-centred type of care management, with few opportunities for direct service development. This is not, however, interpreted negatively by the authors. In complex health and social care communities, it is arguable that this coordinating role is a positive development which legitimately sits alongside extended casework.

In terms of the choice of methods of intervention which social workers may use, the Department of Health's performance indicators for 2004–6 prioritise intensive task-centred involvement:

- 70 per cent of assessments of older people to be completed within two weeks and all completed within four weeks and all assessments to begin within 48 hours of first contact
- all services to be provided within four weeks and 70 per cent within two weeks
- by March 2006, 30 per cent of all older people receiving support to be in receipt of intensive care packages in the community.

Formal expectations of service delivery thus more clearly direct the content of practice than in 1993, and the emphasis on rapid assessment will detract even more from proper monitoring and reviewing functions within care management. It will also further extend the proceduralisation and commodification of the social work labour process, in the shift towards new managerialism (Howe, 1994). It also encapsulates the belief that social problems of isolation, dependency and disability can be solved by the better management of resources and that the process of care management can be described in a cohesive way (Gorman and Postle, 2003). Lymbery (1998) similarly describes the simplistic nature of much care management practice, where the categorisation of need is followed by the delivery of a standardised service response, as an insufficient response to the complexity of human experience. What he does highlight, however, are the opportunities that still exist for social workers to engage with clients away from the direct scrutiny of managers. Even though professionalism may be curtailed with rules and procedures laid down by management, the fact that much social work still takes place in private places means that considerable discretion is still possible.

In a survey of social workers' career patterns conducted in 1993–4, Lyons et al. (1995) found that social workers' reactions to recent changes in their working patterns were closely related to their work settings. A feeling that social work was being fragmented was widespread, leading to an inability on the part of social workers to define and have control over their work. The overall experience of change as positive was related to:

- membership of an autonomous and reasonably well-resourced team with a specific remit, such as HIV/AIDS
- working in a local authority where political values were consistent with the worker's own values
- working in a rural area where community links and networks were more easily developed and maintained
- recent, relevant training or a background in finance or development work.

A willingness to see oneself as a change agent and push forward new ideas was a positive view of community care which was also related to job satisfaction.

A more recent study by Webb and Levin (2000) analysed the impact of the community care changes on social work practice and like Weinberg et al. (2003) found continuities as well as change. The basic concept of community care – enabling people to live in the community as a primary choice – received strong support, and although some social workers commented on the devaluing of their skills, more emphasised the continuing relevance of communication and listening skills in particular. There was evidence, however, that the emphasis had shifted from 'good' practice to accountable practice; there had been an increase in paperwork and new skills in using computers and in financial management, but a loss of role in terms of counselling skills, and also in outreach and groupwork skills. In terms of time spent in face-to-face contact with clients, the *quantity* of time had not changed greatly since 1993, being about one-fifth of the daily workload. *How* the time was spent had changed, with a greater emphasis on assessment as a service in its own right. Hospital social workers also reported a fast turnover of work, because of the more complex interfaces between health and social care. Liaison with health colleagues featured significantly for all social workers, with 90 per cent having daily face-to-face or telephone contact with at least one health professional. Contacts with the Benefits Agency (as it was then) were also significant – almost half of all social workers having contact on welfare rights issues. In terms of unmet need, the findings from this piece of research are significant; 31 per cent of social workers were unable to provide at least one type of support assessed as needed. The complexity of the mixed economy of care was illustrated by the finding that 47 per cent of assessments resulted in care packages using more than one type of sector.

Developments in Scotland

Since the advent of devolution in Scotland in 1998, divergence from policy in England has developed quickly and this has had an impact on the organisation and practice of community care (Valios and Sale, 2003). In Scotland, free personal care in people's own homes as well as in residential settings was introduced in July 2002, whereas in England, only nursing care provided by a registered nurse is free. Curtice and Petch (2002) attribute such divergence to a different value and attitude base in Scotland, with more marked support for public spending. Research by Stalker and Campbell (2002), reviewing care management in Scotland, found that only one authority was using the 'role' model of care management, in 22 it was a 'task' model and 10 authorities reported a mixture of role and task; however, the vast majority of care managers were social work trained, still with a distinctive professional identity. Another issue that has been played out in Scotland is the question of whether care management should be a universal system for cases at all levels of complexity, or whether it is a method of working that should be reserved for only the most intensive cases. The Scottish Executive (2000) picked up this latter definition, reframing care management as *intensive* care management, akin to extended psychosocial casework targeted at people with complex, frequent or rapidly changing needs. However, although 67 per cent of the sample in Stalker and Campbell's research described their cases as 'intensive', few of the service managers saw targeting as an aim of care management, and there was significant diversity in the size and complexity of caseloads. Also, in terms of the purity of models of care management as stages or processes, only a minority of authorities fully separated assessment from care provision, thus showing the extent to which the purchaser/provider split had been undermined over time. There was also a lack of clarity about how and when monitoring should take place. A need for a sound infrastructure in terms of IT, financial information and accounting systems was apparent. One thing that remained constant was an acknowledgement of the importance of interpersonal skills, even within an overtly bureaucratic process.

Skills training in community care

An alternative to seeing care management as a new role or task in social work is to see it as an innovative method of working to be used as an intervention of choice. Superficially, this argument might be attractive because there are many features which care management has in common with traditional social casework, in its emphasis on assessment, care planning, implementing, monitoring and reviewing as part of an individual care plan. To equate care management with social casework is, however, to divorce both from their historical context. As Simiç (1996, p. 13) points out:

> it is not the method that distinguishes care management from casework, it is the social and economic context in which it is employed and the way its resources, intellectual, emotional and material, are developed.

Biggs (1991) sees much of care management as ultimately unworkable because it views interpersonal relationships as unproblematic; it is therefore fatally dismissive of a major method in social work practice – the psychodynamic. Anyone who has worked with carers under stress against a background of difficult family relationships going back over a number of years knows this to be true, and this is the focus of Hughes' (1993) work on the assessment of elderly people in the community and Parker's (1993) study of disability in marriage. To regard such problems of living as purely practical is to throw expensive resources at problems which they will not be able to resolve. Yet it is a common fault of social work practice, particularly in assessment, to oversimplify problems in this way (Ellis, 1993).

The skills required of social workers in community care are a mixture of the old and the new. Smale and Tuson (1993) begin from the premise that there are particular skills that social workers need if their goal is not to be 'expert professionals' but facilitators of full participation in the way in which assessments are carried out. This includes skills in the process of assessment, involving complex negotiations based on:

- expertise in facilitating people's attempts to articulate and identify their own needs and clarify what they want
- sensitivity to language, cultural, racial and gender differences
- the ability to help people through major transitions involving loss
- the ability to negotiate and conciliate between people who have different perceptions, values, attitudes, expectations, wants and needs.

All these things are major attributes of the social work task, and this has led Sheppard (1995) to see social workers as particularly well suited to carrying out the tasks of care management. The importance of interpersonal skills is acknowledged by one of the founders of community care practice; Challis (1992, p. 118) challenges the view that community care is concerned simply with the efficiency of systems and, looking back over the historical development of community care projects, notes that:

> The experimental inputs of the most successful projects were ideational as well as structural. They were substantially about commitments, values and skills. What the structures (including the resources) were intended to do was to enable and encourage people to apply the commitments, values and skills of the new community care philosophy; that is, provide the incentives and rewards which harness individual motivations to achieve the equity and efficiency goals of public policy.

The medium through which services are to be delivered within community care is 'the package of care'. To what extent is this also an innovation? Smale and Tuson (1993, p. 26) emphasise that in care management, as elsewhere, 'social services and social work intervention are a response to the nature of a person's social relationships'; thus the relevant assessment is not that of individuals, but of social relationships. They point out that, for most people, the rudiments of a package of care already exist in the form of support provided by family, neighbours and involved professionals such as the GP. The basic task then is to resolve 'who does what with whom' and 'who is responsible for what', all of which involve skills in negotiation, conflict management and weaving together formal and informal care. Smale and Tuson (p. 33) see such work as having four different components:

- *Direct work* – work with individuals and their immediate families and network to tackle problems which directly affect them
- *Indirect work* – work with wider community groups and other agencies to tackle problems which affect a range of people (including the individuals involved in direct work)
- *Service delivery* – work which involves the maintenance of certain social situations to avoid further distress or institutionalisation, by the provision of services
- *Change agent activities* – work done to effect change in the ways people relate to each other, ways which precipitate or perpetuate social problems of family groups or at community levels.

Care management thus embraces both the social casework approach of traditional social work with individuals and the development role of community social work. It also has both a maintenance component and a change agent component. Care management, if placed in this community context by the breadth of opportunity that it presents, is an exciting and radical new form of work. It requires social workers to think beyond the individual case and confront a commonality of social problems.

User satisfaction

What sort of skills do service users want from social workers under community care? The answer is similar to earlier surveys of satisfaction and dissatisfaction with social work, in that service users want workers who combine practical help with an empathetic approach (Sainsbury, 1975). Early studies of consumer reactions to assessment in community care were undertaken by Age Concern (1994), Age Concern, Scotland (Robertson, 1995) and Mencap (1995). All emphasise the importance of the personal but professional qualities of reliability, empathy, good listening skills and efficiency; these qualities were more important than the professional qualification of the person concerned. The user groups surveyed were realistic (if cynical) about the amount of service that would be provided; one participant in the Age Concern, Scotland research took a view of service provision that became the title of the whole report *Fed and Watered*, protesting at how demeaning it was to be told that needs had been satisfied, provided that the person receiving the service had been 'fed and watered'. However, there was also a strong message in this research that fundamental needs – the need for adequate warmth, an adequate income and a telephone – had to be met before care management at an individual level could make an impact on people's lives. There was a strong expressed need for information on services available, particularly in the Mencap research. The views of service users on community care priorities and worker preferences have remained remarkably stable over time; Vernon and Qureshi (2000), in a survey of disabled service users, found that the way in which services are delivered was seen as an important aspect of empowerment. Service users' own priorities were personal cleanliness and comfort and free movement at home and outside the home. They emphasised user control, staff competence, waiting times, information to support choice and value for money. The major conflicts were between professional and user definitions of independence; the former seeing independence as self-sufficiency and the latter, independence in terms of user control. Independent living was seen as being about access to and control of services enabling individuals to pursue their own lifestyle, while providers tended to prioritise personal care over social support.

The Statement of Expectations

The most important statement of service user priorities is contained in the Statement of Expectations which is an appendix to the *National Occupational Standards for Social Work* (TOPSS, 2002). Derived from consultations with users and carers, the expectation is that social workers in their practice should adhere to the qualities and practices stated below unless there is some specific reason not to do so. The expectations are:

- *Communication skills and information-sharing*: social workers must explain their role and the purpose of contact and their powers including their legal powers; they should be honest if they cannot offer the resources needed, listen actively and share records.
- *Good social work practice*: timekeeping, respect for confidentiality and recognition of the expertise of users and carers are essential features of good practice. Beyond the individual relationship, social workers should link users and carers to support groups and networks and involve users and carers in all meetings which may affect them.
- *Advocacy skills*: not only advice about independent advocacy but also an ability to challenge their own organisation on behalf of users and carers and challenge poor practice, acknowledging when external support is needed.
- *Working with other professionals*: an understanding of what other information different organisations can contribute and how much of this can be shared with users and carers.
- *Knowledge of relevant services* provided by other organisations, benefits and direct payments and legislation.
- *Values of respect, empowerment, honesty and respect for confidentiality*, together with an ability to challenge discriminatory images and practices.

Carers' issues

The vast majority of people providing social care are unpaid and untrained – they are families, friends or neighbours – and the majority will continue to care without any official involvement whatsoever. Indeed, the system of community care is built on there being such a group of people able and willing to provide assistance. Such people may often be grouped together as carers. 'Carer' is a term which covers a range of social situations and should be used with caution for a number of reasons:

- the amount and type of assistance that people provide varies widely and therefore results in qualitatively different situations. These different situations may become unhelpfully muddled by the use of the generic term 'carer'
- the word 'carer' may carry unhelpful and inaccurate connotations of dependency in a relationship
- 'caring for' is, in this way, given a status that 'caring about' does not receive, even though caring about may, in the context of a relationship, be the more important role.

Social workers may relate to carers in a number of different ways: as colleagues, significant others in a relationship with the cared-for person, or service users in their own right. The first approach is based on partnership principles, the second on ideas derived from psychotherapy and the third on citizenship and legalism (Twigg, 1989). Public perceptions of caring may however differ from those of professionals; in Neill and Williams' (1992) study of hospital discharge, for example, a number of interviewees shrank from the application of the term 'carers' to them, seeing it as carrying connotations of obligation and responsibility. A distinction between *carers* (most often family members), who perform intimate physical tasks and whose input of time and energy is substantial, and *supporters* (often friends and neighbours), who do not become involved in physical care but may do practical tasks such as shopping or housework, may therefore be more useful. Caring itself arises in a variety of different family situations. Caring for elderly parents is often seen in terms of duty, although there is no legal obligation to care for parents in old age. Such care therefore lacks the legal foundation that parental care for children has. Caring within marriage has been studied by Parker (1993). Such caring may evolve over a period of time as one partner becomes more frail; in other cases, the sudden onset of disability may provoke a crisis in the marriage. Caring for people with physical needs is also qualitatively different from caring for people with mental health problems, whose needs may fluctuate over time and involve supervision and concern rather than direct help. In a study of family attitudes towards responsibility for their members, Finch and Mason (1993) found that 'being deserving' rated highly in legitimising care by others. There is also a tendency for other family members to withdraw once one person is identified as a main carer.

Although spouse carers are almost as likely to be men as women (Arber and Gilbert, 1993), Finch (1989), writing from a feminist perspective, is critical of the extent to which community care is predicated on the labour of women, particularly as women are also assumed to have the major responsibility for the care of children. Suggestions of a return to communal or institutional care are resisted by Morris (1993), who sees such a movement as divisive and discriminatory against disabled women. Less emphasis on 'care' and more on 'enabling' would seek to remove the negative connotations of exploitation and dependency.

'Caring about' as a replacement for the notion of 'caring for' humanises the situation being described and gives it dignity. The situation of children who care for adults in the same household is, for example, often interpreted narrowly as caring for, with concerns focused on the appropriateness, or otherwise, of the tasks that the child is undertaking, and on the abrogation of the parental role. A more positive approach is to discuss each of the participants' feelings about the situation; there may be a good deal of caring about going on, with the child wishing to contribute to the household, and the parent concerned for and involved in the emotional development of the child (SSI, 1996b).

The task for the social worker is to perceive how the system itself works; what sustains the carer/cared-for relationship and what undermines it. Qureshi et al. (1983) propose that helping in its widest sense is characterised by exchange theory, in other words, people will calculate (consciously or not) whether what they gain from the relationship, in terms of satisfaction or reward, is worth the physical or emotional effort they put into it. As the balance will be different for each individual and will change over time, exchanges need to be carefully monitored and, where necessary, supported. It is important that local authority eligibility criteria are designed with the needs of carers in mind. A breakdown in the caring/supporting relationship is a more potent factor than the level of disability in precipitating admission to residential care (Warburton, 1989). Research by Levin et al. (1989) has found that daycare and respite care services are highly valued by carers of older people, enabling them to carry on caring for longer. Nevertheless, social workers must be sensitive to a desire by carers to use such services to begin the process of disengagement from caring; not to be explicit about the purpose for which such services are being used means that social workers and carers may be working to different agendas.

The Carers and Disabled Children Act 2000 gives carers of adults and disabled children a right to assessment, even if the person for whom they provide care is refusing assessment. It also enables local authorities to provide carers services directly to carers, or offer direct payments for the purchase of services. Thus it gives carers a status in their own right, independently of the person for whom they care. Information about the availability of assessments is important for the success of any carers policy. Research by Arksey et al. (2000), into the working of the predecessor 1995 Carers (Recognition and Services) Act, found that knowledge of the Act was limited; around half of all carers interviewed did not realise they had received an assessment, and carers were not routinely provided with a written record of outcomes. Similarly, Robinson and Williams' (2002) research into carers of people with learning disabilities found that the 1995 Act was not widely used or understood by this group of carers. Greater involvement from health and housing services and responsiveness to changes in carers' circumstances were identified as improvements to current practice. Support for carers is higher now on the social policy agenda, with grant aid available to develop carers services. The social construction of different carers' identities has led Stalker (2003) to conclude that at the end of a decade of community care, carers have increasingly been treated as service providers in their own right (as well as recipients of services) and that, to some extent, informal caring has, in line with Twigg's typology, become professionalised.

Carers will have other demands on their time and demographic changes have meant that there are more people in the community in need of support, but also more women in the employment market carrying multiple roles. Section 8 of the Employment Relations Act 1999 gives employees the right to a reasonable amount of time off as unpaid leave to provide assistance to 'dependants', or to deal with unexpected disruptions to their care. Some employers give more generous opportunities for leave to carers within family-friendly policies. Phillips et al. (2002) investigated the experiences of carers of older adults in the light of such policies. They found that although 1 in 10 employees were involved in caring for parents or parents-in-law, there was a lack of openness about these caring responsibilities compared to childcare responsibilities. This has led to very few employees taking advantage of policies that identified them as 'in need' or 'not coping'. Phillips et al. concluded that there remains an urgent need for employers to address these issues if they are to have a sustainable workforce in the longer term.

Social networks

The interlocking nature of individual and collective responses to the problem of need was identified in the Barclay Report (1982). SSDs were seen as having failed to come up with strategies for linking statutory and non-statutory sources of care provision into a coherent plan. Community care planning enables, indeed requires, such a strategy to take place. It is the responsibility not only of departments but also of individual social workers to develop skills in 'exploring communities of interest which may be important to a particular client' (Barclay Report, para. 3.30). For care management to operate properly, it is important not only that individuals' needs are understood, but that individuals, groups and organisations within communities are prepared and able to provide the facilities needed (Coulshed and Orme, 1998). The theoretical base is close to that of radical social work, with its emphasis on collective action and a perception of individual problems as political issues. This is not to deny, however, that networks may have a therapeutic role to play as change agents in finding solutions to the problems of individuals and families.

Seed (1990) sees individuals as having networks which comprise layers of close or more distant social involvement (see Figure 7.1). The analysis of networking in social support systems has developed from systems theory, and offers a way of exploring how people's social networks operate in ways that help or hamper their ability to cope in the community. Network analysis has been successfully used to assist people with learning disabilities to move out of hospital care into the community; the role of the social worker being variously that of counsellor, mediator, planner or advocate (Atkinson, 1986). Its value to social workers is as a tool for understanding the social experiences of clients and composing a picture of the informal support systems that may need to be mobilised or even created (Reigate, 1997). A network might include close relatives, neighbours and friends, voluntary helpers, people with similar problems coming together in a self-help group and members of formal organisations like churches or trade unions. Seed (1990) suggests that keeping a networking diary is a useful tool for maintaining

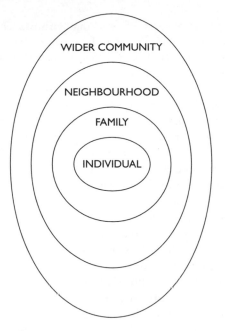

Figure 7.1 Social networks

the client as the focus of planning and illustrating the client's own ability to form networks in the community.

Smale and Tuson (1993, p. 40) see social workers as being proactive in making community resources available:

> Care managers will have to work in partnership with local people to negotiate the need for, plan, initiate, support, sustain and maintain local groups, voluntary organisations and schemes for meeting certain people's needs.

This echoes Goldberg and Warburton's (1979) conclusions, from their study of social work in the aftermath of the Seebohm reorganisation in the early 1970s, that rather than occasional routine visits, the relief of isolation and loneliness, help with small chores and emotional and practical support to informal carers would need to be provided by volunteers or 'good neighbours', under the sponsorship of either the statutory or voluntary sector. Similar convictions as to the appropriateness of and capacity for developing community support systems were behind an innovative community care project in Kent (Davies and Challis, 1986), which provided the research evidence for the development of community care (see Chapter 2). In this project, local people with no previous caring experience were recruited to perform routine domiciliary tasks for frail older people and their main carers.

Finding, supporting and sustaining networks within a community can be a major part of the social work task. Also acknowledged is the fact that individuals, agencies, volunteers, community resources and other professionals within a network may have differing perspectives. Working with difference (Home Office,

1995) is thus an important aspect of working within a community; structural factors such as gender, race and class may be more powerful in themselves than the inclusive idea of community. It is also necessary to acknowledge that people may have different motivations on a personal level for giving time, money and expertise to assist others, and that these need to be supported (Qureshi et al., 1983). Some people may need time from the worker, some may need financial reward, while some may simply need acknowledgement that they are doing a good job. Although volunteering is often seen as an individual activity, it can also be organised collectively through self-help organisations and community groups, and may include people who are service users in their own right (Payne, 1995). Volunteering England was created in April 2004 as a national volunteer development agency organised regionally to bring more coherence to volunteering (see www.volunteering.org.uk). Developments such as a youth volunteering strategy, supported by a mentor system, are likely future innovations. The strategy will be aimed both at students and those seeking to enter the job market. Again, social workers will have to contribute positively to exchanges in the relationship, not simply take the benefit of the volunteer's time.

Payne (1995) explores the difference between community development work and community work. Community development work is based on pluralism – the idea that formal authorities, although they have an important role in providing services and taking a lead in planning, are not the only bodies concerned with public welfare. Voluntary organisations and neighbourhood groups will play a significant role in developing a truly local response to need. The basic tenets of community development are therefore highly congruent with those of community care, although, as Payne points out (p. 169):

> The central conflict within community development is that between developing services and projects which respond to social services requirements, and promoting involvement in processes for community decision-making among people in particular areas or with shared interests, which may not reflect or may conflict with social services priorities . . . A distinction must also be drawn between the interests of the community as a whole and those of users and carers. There may be no interest in the particular needs of groups of users of community care services; priorities with other people may lie elsewhere.

Community development work is essentially proactive in developing community awareness as well as services or facilities, such as luncheon clubs or sitting services, so that carers can meet together. The role of the paid worker becomes one of a facilitator rather than a leader. Local groups, based around a common interest, can be helped to grow, enabled to use community facilities such as village halls or be given help in developing businesslike tasks such as running a meeting or organising a budget. The most famous account of community social work in action is the 'patch' system in Normanton, Wakefield, described by Hadley and McGrath (1984). Social workers working on a patch within a closely defined geographical area would acquire on the ground information about the local area, develop an accessibility to local people and forge strong personal links with other professionals in the area such as GPs, community nurses, representatives of voluntary organisations and churches. Community social work, as endorsed in the Barclay Report (1982) and by Payne (1995), would be judged by its effectiveness in terms of its major objectives of involving local people in decision-making and making locally sensitive services available.

Mayo (1994) sees two different perspectives on community work: the technicist and the transformational. The *technicist* promotes community initiatives within the framework of existing social relations, whereas the *transformational* seeks to develop strategies and build alliances for social change. Transformational community work is inherently political, in that it challenges the location of power within officially sanctioned groups. Structural inequalities, poverty and racism are all confronted by community work. In so doing, it exposes the benign assumptions of community care policy that society is based on consensus and formal and informal care can easily be interwoven. Quilgars (2004) has evaluated a community care development project in Hull set up by a partnership of local statutory and voluntary agencies to meet low-level support and care needs in two deprived communities. It was found that community definitions directly influenced the shape and development of the project as the regeneration of community spirit and capacity-building support to local groups and networks. In other words, this was an example of care *by* the community, rather than simply *in* the community. Agencies were willing to try new ways of working where previously they had had little involvement with the community. A key challenge to increasing social capital, however, lay in recruiting and retaining volunteers and reaching more vulnerable groups. Measures of success were on occasions contested, particularly the social model of health promotion adopted by the community and the medical model used by the healthcare services.

The 'community' basis of community care is challenged from a different perspective by Bulmer (1987). Bulmer develops the idea of a community of 'limited liability', based on temporary and highly focused alliances between people who have a common interest, for example in the provision of good quality education for their children at the local school or the building of a bypass to alleviate traffic congestion locally. It cannot be assumed that this community of interest will extend to other matters, particularly as people's major ties remain kinship ties, which survive despite greater social mobility. The isolation and rejection of people with mental health problems or learning disabilities is seen as underlining the point that, in many people's minds, community care means care by the families (if any) of those in need of care, and not some wider conception of social responsibility. The consequence is that formal, statutory sector involvement is necessary to support people who are without family ties. Yet, at the same time, informal care by families alone is not adequate, largely due to the absence of a proper family policy to compensate financially those family members who provide care. Community care policies which ignore these infrastructure issues are therefore built on shaky foundations.

The debate continues as to whether communities are sufficiently self-reliant or internally cohesive to be able to operate autonomously to challenge existing patterns of organisational responsibility. Stewart (2000, p. 23) sees 'communities of place, of background, interest or concern' as all possible and likely ways of being involved in community governance to tackle environmental problems, community safety, discrimination and social exclusion that are difficult for monolithic organisations to manage.

Jordan (2000) also sees a new conception of public social services, more firmly rooted in neighbourhoods and linked with community groups, as a vision for which to strive, but one which is hampered by the penalising through economic policy of informal household work, neighbourliness, volunteering and other communal activities. Social work remains slow to see its development potential in this area; it continues to be true that, as Clarke (2000, p. 1) observes, despite the applicability of the National Occupational Standards to work with communities, 'British social work is the only institution of its kind in Europe which consigns community to the sidelines'.

Concluding comments

This chapter looked at the changing nature of social work practice within community care and the different skills needed to evidence professional competence. Working with individual service users still draws on the enduring skills of psychosocial casework, although opportunities to work face to face may be limited by the new priority given to throughput and coordinating tasks. Community care has, however, given opportunities, as yet unfulfilled, to extend the community basis of social work practice in tackling social exclusion and working to the agendas set by service users and carers themselves.

PAUSE AND REFLECT

Construct a diagram to illustrate the social network of a person who you know (or one of your own social network). What are the significant individuals and organisations within this network?

CASE STUDY

Collaboration

Polly Richards is 35 years old and lives alone in her flat on a local authority housing estate. She has a diagnosis of schizophrenia and receives fortnightly visits from a community mental health nurse (CMHN). Polly rarely leaves her flat, except to visit the local shops and café. The CMHN has become concerned that local youths are visiting Polly's flat when they are supposed to be at school. Small amounts of money and some possessions have gone missing. Polly has said that she enjoyed their company at first, but now she feels harassed by them. She has asked them to stay away, but they have not done so.

The CMHN asks your advice on what to do about this situation. What would you advise?

FURTHER READING

Fook, J. (2002) *Social Work: Critical Theory and Practice*. London: Sage.
Explores, from a critical postmodern social work perspective, the implications of managerialism ousting professional discourses in social work.

Jordan, B. with Jordan, C. (2000) *Social Work and the Third Way: Tough Love as Social Policy*. London: Sage.
Based on a wealth of personal experience, the authors analyse the actual and potential role of the social worker in society. The use of social work as an instrument for realising New Labour policies is explored in context. An alternative vision of public social services more firmly rooted in neighbourhoods and linked with community groups is proposed, set against a critique of current roles in enforcement, surveillance and control.

Trevithick, P. (2000) *Social Work Skills: A Practice Handbook*. Buckingham: Open University Press.
Looks at basic and enduring interviewing, helping and communication skills and a toolbox of interventions needed by the skilled practitioner.

CHAPTER 8

Changing Values

Introduction

Social work practice not only needs a coherent theoretical basis, it also needs to be rooted in a professional values system. The historical development of social work values is explored in this chapter and the GSCC's *Code of Practice for Social Care Workers* (2002) is set out as a necessary standard against which fitness to practice is to be judged. The practical expression of values within community care practice is explored through the meaning of such contested concepts as participation, empowerment, advocacy and anti-discriminatory and anti-oppressive practice.

KEY ROLE 6

Demonstrate professional competence in social work practice

GSCC Code of Practice for Social Workers

Social care workers must:

▶ Protect the rights and promote the interests of service users and carers
▶ Strive to establish and maintain the trust and confidence of service users and carers
▶ Promote the independence of service users while protecting them as far as possible from danger or harm
▶ Respect the rights of service users whilst seeking to ensure that their behaviour does not harm themselves or other people
▶ Uphold public trust and confidence in social care services
▶ Be accountable for the quality of their work and take responsibility for maintaining and improving their knowledge and skills

Knowledge, skills and values

The current requirements for qualification continue to describe social work as a combination of knowledge, skills and values. But it is arguable that no real distinction can be drawn between these three elements of practice (Banks, 2001). Knowledge is rendered sterile by an unskilled application, and what we seek to know – more precisely, how we understand and make sense of what we know – is determined by our value position. The value base of social work is explored here within a framework of community care. Particular attention is paid to social work dilemmas when values conflict, for example when a cared-for person's right to self-determination is in conflict with a carer's need for respite. Three particular areas are chosen for consideration in this chapter in terms of their value base: meeting the needs of black service users; the rights of people with disabilities; and difficulties posed by the onset of mental incapacity.

Values in social work are part of a professionally protected dogma; they are essentially collective and may be in juxtaposition to the personal beliefs of the individual social worker. Social work values are not static; they evolve in line with changes in society and organisations to which social workers must respond. Although the classic social work values of respect for persons and client self-determination still subsist, today they may emerge in a different formulation, as working in partnership and empowerment. The proactive expression of social work's value base is seen in the development of anti-discriminatory and anti-oppressive practice.

Social work practice is in need of a moral base because its concern is with the care and development of vulnerable people. Social workers are called on to make difficult decisions affecting the integrity of families and individuals' freedom to live the life they choose. Social work decisions are 'decisions under uncertainty', which cannot be adjudicated simply by the application of technical or procedural rules (Evans and Harris, 2004). Banks (2001) uses the term 'dilemma' to describe the essentially moral choices that social workers have to make when considering which of two possible outcomes to pursue. Should the social worker, for example, section a person under the Mental Health Act for the protection of the public, or support his or her desire to remain in the community with (possibly inadequate) support? In such a situation, choices should be guided by values, so that hopefully the least detrimental alternative can be achieved.

What are values?

The OED describes values as 'the principles or moral standards of a person or social group'. Values ultimately help to guide action:

> a value is something to do with what you ought to do in practice. This may not be the same as what you want to do or what it is in your interests to do, or in fact what you actually do. (Howe, 1996)

There are also two kinds of values: primary, or intrinsic values, where things are seen as good in their own right; and instrumental values, things that are worth pursuing because of their end result. The difficulty is that none of these things is uncontroversial; people in different cultures and at different points in time will disagree over what primary values are and the authority, religious or secular, from which they stem. Social work, when it emphasises legalism, measured change and control, fits well into a rational view of the world which is essentially that of modernism. The stance of postmodernism is to emphasise the relativity of values; there are no universal standards or laws by which we can understand either human behaviour or society.

Divergence exists not only in the tasks that social workers undertake (Davies, 1997); it exists also in the significance, meaning and value to be given to those actions (Shardlow, 2002). Thus, in discussing anti-oppressive practice, Clifford (1994) emphasises historical and cultural factors which lead to an approach based on social construction theories of oppression. Dominelli (1998) adopts a person-centred philosophy and an egalitarian value system, while Dalrymple and Burke (1995) emphasise reflexivity, requiring that social workers consider the ways in which their own social identity and values affect the information they gather, so that 'the act of challenging' relates to themselves as much as to others and external systems.

The historical development of social work values

The development of value statements for social work was first grounded in the one-to-one casework tradition, with values appropriate to that relationship being propounded most famously by Biestek (1957). Biestek's 'seven principles' are summarised by Banks (2001) as:

1. Individualisation; the recognition of each person's unique qualities
2. The recognition of each person's need to express their own feelings, both positive and negative
3. Controlled emotional involvement
4. Acceptance of people as they really are
5. A non-judgemental attitude; separating out the person from the behaviour
6. User self-determination
7. Confidentiality.

This approach, often condensed into the phrase 'respect for persons', was recognised by Biestek himself to be subject to legal requirements, to a 'higher duty' to self, to other individuals or to the community (Banks, 2001). Controversially, this concept of 'personhood' applied only to people who were capable of rational thought and self-determined action, which in itself has led to difficulties in applying Biestek's principles to people lacking mental capacity (see below). Principles which emphasise the integrity of the social worker–individual relationship are also best suited to a professional model of social work, which sees the social worker as an autonomous professional and the other party as a 'client'. It may be less appropriate where the social worker is an employee of a statutory agency working to a legal mandate. Given that the practice of social work is a socially sanctioned role, other types of ethical principles concerned with utility (promoting the greatest balance of good over evil) and justice (distributing the good(s) as widely and/or fairly as possible) may claim to be more relevant expressions of social work values than simply individualism (Banks, 2001). The hospitalisation of people who are mentally ill (because of the risk they pose to the public, rather than themselves) is justified by utilitarian principles because it is the greatest good for the greatest number. The client in competition for scarce resources becomes a service user – a person in receipt of care according to their assessed ability to pay. In this sense, utilitarian values are easily espoused by community care policy. However, in community care, there is little respect for the concept of distributive justice; on the whole services are not spread thinly amongst those who might derive some benefit from them. The consumer's self-determination is bounded by legal parameters; his or her needs are not expressed in terms of self-actualisation. The emphasis is on process and instrumental values, such as the right to a fair hearing or access to records. The user is treated as an object of concern – a risk to be assessed and later controlled.

A move away from both individualisation and utilitarianism towards a growing awareness of structural oppression, particularly with regard to women and black communities, took place in the late 1980s. A key theme was 'praxis', the notion of committed action in which values are part of a radical challenge to structural inequalities (Banks, 2001). Under such an approach, equal opportunities policies, for example, would be seen as racist for ignoring difference, and the task of the social worker is one of challenging injustice at a structural level. But it is not just about adopting a value position, it is about doing, in particular, making a commitment to the process of connection. In relation to competences, anti-discriminatory practice is about professionals using authority in a way that is helpful for someone less powerful than themselves. In order to achieve this, it is necessary to examine the impact of difference on oneself, use knowledge and research to inform practice, consider the use of language, both orally and in written reports, and critically evaluate both agency policy and procedures.

The use of language is a fundamental indicator of the theoretical position held by the user and is a signpost to the type of practice that will follow. Thus Braye and Preston-Shoot (1995) are able to highlight traditional versus radical values in social care by juxtapositioning, for example, the traditional value of respect for persons with that of citizenship, paternalism and protection with participation, and partnership with empowerment or user control. They perceive social workers as working to either a broadly reformist agenda, where there are equal opportunities to reform the relationship between service providers and users within a social democratic framework, or a radical agenda, where issues of power and oppression are uppermost and an individual's life chances are determined by his or her position in society.

Can the different approaches to values, from individualistic, utilitarian and radical perspectives, be reconciled? Jordan (1995) argues that they cannot, because they are inherently in conflict with each other. Formal, professionally driven statements of values (GSCC, 2002; BASW, 2002) may juxtapose elements from each of these perspectives without acknowledging that the achievement of some is dependent on the destruction of others. As Jordan argues, these same liberal values of choice and privacy are amongst the strongest intellectual defences of the privileges of wealth, whiteness and masculinity on which structural oppression is based. Which values are to take precedence? There is no guidance on this and, arguably, there cannot be, if, as Howe (1996) argues, the task is really to acknowledge the imperfections and compromises, trading and negotiation that inevitably have to take place. This makes difficult, if not impossible, the attainment of any formal view of values as objectively verifiable and hence assessable.

The GSCC's *Code of Practice for Social Care Workers* (2002) is presented as a formal statement of values. All social care workers are expected to meet this code and the GSCC may take formal action in respect of registered workers for failure to do so. Employers are also required to take account of this code in making any decisions about the conduct of their staff. The emphasis within professional training on competences and learning outcomes often disguises the fact that what actually happens in the learning process is not often studied or understood (Yelloly and Henkel, 1995). What develops in the relationship between the individual worker and the agency may itself be explicable in terms of the psychoanalytic concepts of conflict, ambivalence, anxiety and defence. Jones and Joss (1995) consider that the value base of the individual worker may thus include informal rules and meanings which derive from subcultures within the organisation. Bion (1967) also uses psychoanalytic concepts to explain the unconscious and unverbalised feelings of anger or depression that are aroused in workers by the bureaucratisation of the work they are called on to do. Para-doxically, this abrogation of the opportunity for individual development may ultimately work to the detriment of the organisation. Where social workers are sustained and enabled by their organisation to carry out difficult and challenging tasks, the experiences gained foster growth in the organisation. Hence, the capacity for creative individual thought will be weakened by demands that are 'off task', such as apparently meaningless paperwork and sterile meetings, and will be lost altogether if energy is diverted to the construction of 'bad objects' at the level of management or policy-making. The social worker who is asked to assess need without having the resources to meet that need is also likely to suffer (in a personal, psychological sense, as well as a professional sense) from cognitive dissonance, as the gap between aspiration and reality becomes more difficult logically to sustain (Postle, 2002).

Values within community care

Pietroni (1995) analyses the effect that community care changes have had on professionalism and locates such changes within postmodernism. The loss of certainty, acceptance of a relativist philosophy and the fragmentation of values, thoughts and belief are all accepted features of postmodernism. Most important, in terms of social work values, is what is termed 'the waning of affect' – people become 'commodities', 'bits', 'episodes', rather than significant individuals. Specifically in relation to community care, cultural change has been highlighted by the adoption of market mechanisms, which in turn has led to (Pietroni, 1995, p. 45):

- The commodification of care through needs assessment, care packaging and care management
- The emphasis on audit, information and databases, especially to serve the welfare exchange market structured around the purchaser/provider split. Knowledge and information in this way themselves become marketable commodities

- The near disappearance of the term 'social work' without official acknowledgement in the glossaries and directories accompanying the NHSCCA 1990
- A world where the term 'quality' can in effect mean *quantity* of care provided. If care management is defined by resource-based eligibility criteria, care management as a process can also mean managing the lack of care
- The rhetoric of 'user-centred seamless service' and 'partnership', with a seductive undertow that evokes sentimentality in the place of a more rational appraisal of the viability of new policies, given the existing resource framework
- The constant change of senior managers and organisational structures leading to an absence of authoritative leadership.

The adoption of agency values as taken-for-granted expressions of the common good is also problematic, insofar as it subordinates individual thought to organisational culture. The legitimacy of such definitions is accepted by the GSCC in the requirement to uphold public trust and confidence in social care services. Similarly, the fourth requirement of the code of practice that 'social care workers will respect the rights of service users whilst seeking to ensure that their behaviour does not harm themselves or other people' is to be seen in the context of more prescriptive control over people's behaviour, following the introduction of devices such as antisocial behaviour orders and supervised discharge of mental health patients. Furthermore, the emphasis within the code of practice is on equal opportunities rather than on either social inclusion or critical social work practice, in the sense of anti-oppressive action (Fook, 2002).

Are there positive elements of community care which relate to values, an understanding of which supports good practice? The areas which best promote change in community care are seen by Shardlow (2002) as participation, empowerment, advocacy and anti-discriminatory and anti-oppressive practice:

- *Participation* may be said to be based on traditional Kantian principles of respect for persons; involving people in planning and decision-making is inherently respectful and can be a source of personal growth
- *Empowerment* is more than an instrumental value that enables people to make choices; insofar as it asserts the sovereignty of the decision-maker, it is a primary value of citizenship
- *Advocacy* is instrumental in a utilitarian sense by emphasising distributive justice and fair treatment for all and a (potentially at least) equal entitlement to bid for goods on offer
- *Anti-discriminatory and anti-oppressive practice* positively promote difference as part of an agenda for change.

Thus the historical development of the value base of social work from the individual to the structural can be seen to come together within community care, as long as the practitioner remains aware of the different sources on which such practice is based.

Participation

Participation by service users in the design and delivery of services was heralded in the Foreword to the Griffiths Report (1988) as a basic cornerstone of community care policy:

> The whole thrust of my work has been to ensure a move from an administered paternalistic provision of service to a managed system of meeting consumer needs in a way which will provide a quality of service economically and effectively delivered and involving and motivating both the consumer and the staff.

Croft and Beresford (1990) identified two competing philosophies underpinning user involvement: consumerism and self-advocacy. Consumerism was defined as the seeking of information from users by agencies that wish to improve their efficiency, economy and effectiveness. Agencies do this primarily in order to find solutions to their own problems, such as, is their product the one that the consumer wants? By contrast, self-advocacy is user-driven, and here the aim is empowerment. An example of consumerism would be advisory committees set up under the Care Standards Act 2000 to comment on the registration process, while an example of self-advocacy would be the setting up of carers forums specifically to raise awareness of the needs and rights of carers. Agencies should therefore clarify from the beginning what kind of involvement is being sought and what commitment can be given to act on what people say they want. There is also an important role for service users in setting the research agenda and being directly involved in the dissemination of research findings; a stage beyond service delivery and evaluation. The SCIE (2004) accordingly sets out principles for effective user participation in social care, in the context of commissioning research to evaluate the impact that user participation has had on the design and delivery of services – an impact which has yet to be explored.

Empowerment

Shardlow (2002) observes the term 'empowerment' as being used in the literature in two different ways. He sees Stevenson and Parsloe's (1993) definition of empowerment in community care as being centred on the articulation and meeting of social care needs, while Braye and Preston-Shoot (1995) emphasise both the developmental nature of empowerment – extending one's ability to take effective decisions – and its role in maximising people's quality of life, by enabling disempowered people to have a greater voice in institutions, services and situations which affect them in the attainment of their own goals.

Hoyes et al. (1993) have produced a 'ladder of empowerment' to measure the extent to which users both individually and collectively have the power to take decisions or influence the decision-making process. The 'top' of the ladder reflects the highest level of empowerment, and the bottom of the ladder is the lowest (Hoyes et al., 1993).

HIGH   Users have the authority to take all decisions
           Users have the authority to take selected decisions
           Users' views are sought before decisions are finalised
           Users may take the initiative to influence decisions
           Decisions are publicised and explained before implementation
LOW   Information is given about decisions made

Jack (1995, p. 6) is sceptical of claims that empowerment can be achieved through participation in service planning and poses the question: 'Do participation and involvement "empower" service users or is their involvement itself potentially disempowering through absorption, colonisation or the bureaucratic dissipation of legitimate protest?' Real empowerment involves control – over money and over resources – and is essentially a political activity. It is not something which is in the gift of professionals; it is something which arises from the demands of individuals or groups to have their needs met. The model of care management which best fits the idea of empowerment is that of service brokerage (Brandon and Towell, 1989). In this model, the care manager acts as an agent of the service user and/or their family to commission services from a variety of sources which fit the agenda which he or she is given. The care manager has no resources of his or her own, but negotiates for individualised funding to obtain services that the user needs and wants. Thus, it is the service user and not the professional who sets the agenda.

Jack (1995) contrasts empowerment and enablement; terms which are often confused in social work parlance. *Empowerment* involves establishing the legitimacy of user-determined goals as an attribute of citizenship. *Enablement* is not a political concept, however, but a professional skill. In the context of community care, the professional may involve a user in the assessment process for a service; the worker may thus 'enable' the user to develop self-confidence, self-esteem and negotiation skills through this process. However, the power to purchase that service and withdraw it is retained by the professional who has given over none of the power to control the process or its outcome (Jack, 1995, p. 11). In its proper sense, empowerment, by contrast, is about having access to decision-making processes which have the rights of users at their centre, and therefore has a strong procedural aspect.

Advocacy

'Protect the rights and promote the interests of service users and carers' is the first requirement of the GSCC code of practice for social care workers. How feasible is it for workers to undertake such a task through the use of advocacy within an administrative or entrepreneurial system of care management? Advocacy is 'speaking on behalf of' another, usually in a formal and often in a quasi-legal context. In contrast with empowerment, advocacy does not give power, it gives the right to make representations to those (others) who have the power. It implies partisanship; a sense of belonging to the person on whose behalf the advocacy is taking place. It is unlikely that anyone who is an employee of the agency which makes the final decision on the granting of resources or the settlement of a dispute concerning property, money or even individual liberty can properly be said to be acting as an advocate. The *Practitioners' Guide* (SSI/DoH, 1991, para. 74) recognises this: 'the devolution of responsibility to allocate resources changes the nature of the relationship between practitioner and user. Practitioners are less able to act as advocates on users' behalf.' This highlights the need to develop opportunities for independent representation and advocacy in parallel with care management arrangements.

Harding and Beresford (1996, p. 30) find evidence that advocacy is seen by service users and carers as an important service: 'Advocacy is crucial to express their wants and needs, their preferences and anxieties, their complaints and objections' – a fact that is not reflected in what health and local authorities choose to fund. Payne (1995) distinguishes different types of advocacy:

- *Citizen advocacy* which operates on a one-to-one basis with one person representing the views of another, usually in a formal setting such as a case conference or review
- *Self-advocacy* in which training and support may be provided to enable people to represent themselves assertively
- *Group advocacy* which brings together a number of people with similar interests who operate as a group to represent their shared interests.

The first two are essentially individual and operate on a case-by-case basis. Advising and assisting a mentally ill person to present an appeal against compulsory detention for treatment at a mental health review tribunal is one example of direct advocacy which a social worker could perform or for which agencies can fund voluntary organisations to provide training. The third is directed not so much to individual change but structural change. The power of the group is also greater than the sum of its parts. Group advocacy may in some circumstances become community action when sufficient people are involved. Group advocacy may be seen as the preferred method if the aim is for the group to become involved in service delivery decisions and reframe how the group itself is perceived. This type of advocacy may thus be seen as cause advocacy rather than case advocacy (Rees, 1991). Representative advocacy of vulnerable adults is high on the legal as well as the social policy agenda, in relation to mental health and learning disability and other adults lacking capacity, and is likely to be enshrined in legislation in these areas.

Anti-discriminatory and anti-oppressive practice

Braye and Preston-Shoot (1995) contrast anti-discriminatory practice and anti-oppressive practice. They see the former as a non-radical value which locates challenges to both personal and structural inequalities within equal opportunities policies based on voluntary change. By contrast, anti-oppressive practice places less confidence on the value of remedial action in changing a service user's experience of oppression when such oppression is endemic to the whole fabric of society:

Thus, while personal and organisational action for equality is important, its focus must be wider than merely the relationship created through use of services if equality is to be addressed on a significant scale. (Braye and Preston-Shoot, 1995, p. 43)

Dominelli (1998) sees anti-oppressive practice as a normal part of citizenship entitlements valuing difference, whilst refusing to recognise a hierarchy of oppressions within race, gender, age or disability. Adams (1998) sees anti-oppressive practice as a collectivist professional approach to oppression and contrasts it with empowerment, which is the achievement of powers from professionals by individual service users. In this sense, anti-oppressive practice is a manifestation of a radical alternative value base which is inherently political (Thompson, 1993).

Different discourses may be in conflict in relation to contemporary social work values. Dominelli (2002, p. 118) sees the human rights agenda as an important focus of concern for anti-oppressive social work practice, which links the individual with their social and physical environment: 'In this process of change for social work, values should be visualised as dynamic entities rather than as fixed and immutable objects.' Clarke (2000) sees the ethics of practice as being influenced also by a discourse of regulation and personal accountability. He does not present this in terms of conflict, however, but in terms of assimilation, emphasising the function of social work as an aspect of public policy, within which 'the ethics of practice must take fully into account the political issues and choices built in to professional principles and agency structures'. The content of social work ethics is not thus solely for the profession to determine; it is governed by the political climate within which social workers work. Jordan (2000) quotes Driver and Martell (1997) as seeing this climate as conformist, conservative, prescriptive, moral and concerned with individual responsibility. This is manifested in benefits and services that were formerly entitlements becoming conditional privileges; standardised services being tailored to individual needs only through close assessment processes and targeting services on those most at risk or dangerous to others (Jordan, 2000). This raises doubts as to

whether professional social work any longer seeks to be credible at street level, with service users and carers, or whether it is developing an arm's length, office-based, report-writing, official kind of practice which leaves face-to-face work to others. (Jordan, 2000, p. 37)

Values in practice

Has community care made ethically sensitive social work more difficult to achieve in practice? Jack (1995) argues that the introduction of market principles, against the background of a breakdown in consensus about the size and function of the welfare state, has necessarily had an effect on the profession of social work, and, in particular:

Any claims still made to moral integrity based on professional vocation and the primacy of the client's interests are seen to be increasingly suspect as the difference between the caring professions and other businesses become less and less apparent. (Jack, 1995, p. 3)

'People work' as Thompson (2003) explains, so often involves the exercise of power, frequently with relatively powerless people. For this reason, it is important that the worker acts positively to promote equality, rather than exacerbate the inequalities that exist in society and in people's lives. Language is important, as discourse embeds discriminatory ideas into everyday relationships and activities. Each piece of work undertaken should therefore be evaluated, according to Thompson (2003), in terms of:

- The extent to which issues of social location and discrimination were taken account of at a personal, cultural and structural level
- The extent to which we acted in partnership
- Whether our actions were appropriate in the circumstances
- Lessons to be learned, in terms of pitfalls and strengths.

Thus anti-oppressive practice is a standard against which actions and interventions can be evaluated as well as a theory for understanding. The extent to which community care policies acknowledge and respect difference is crucial for the ability of individual practitioners to practice in an anti-oppressive way.

Working with black service users

Services for people from black and minority ethnic groups are a generally underdeveloped area of community care; recognition of structural issues may be further undermined by traditional divisions between user groups which ignore commonalties of interest, for example amongst black service users of childcare as well as adult services. The White Paper *Community Care in the Next Decade and Beyond* (DoH, 1989b) acknowledges that 'good community care must recognise the circumstances of minority communities, be sensitive to their needs and be planned in consultation with them'. No further guidance, however, is given on how this is to be achieved. Cameron et al. (1996) consider that the system of community care may create further disadvantages for black and ethnic minority groups because of the tendency to individualise problems and because services are organised according to white norms.

Heavy reliance is placed on the voluntary sector to make specialist provision, which can lead to marginalisation, particularly if such services are short term and inadequately funded. The values upon which assessments are based may be inappropriate – a particular example is the assumption that independence from the family is to be encouraged.

Ahmad and Atkin (1996) take this argument further by emphasising the pervasiveness of racist attitudes, which may lead on to health and social problems being defined in terms of cultural deficits, particularly in the mental health field. Certainly, Norman (1980) exposed the 'triple jeopardy' facing older women growing old in a second homeland; they were identifiable as the group least likely to receive appropriate psychiatric treatment and care. Access to services – being aware of what is available and how to use it – is poor (Atkin and Rollings, 1993). Ahmad and Atkin see community care positively as an opportunity for new forms of provision to arise, but according to them (1996, p. 6):

> A challenge for academics and practitioners alike, including in relation to community care, is to recognise the context of black people's lives, to which their cultural norms, values and resources and racialised oppression and marginalisation are equally pertinent.

Community care policies which give limited attention to structural factors will thus provide an inadequate basis for service provision.

Burke and Harrison (2002) look outside the individual service user/worker relationship to the way in which the team and the agency have their work prioritised and constrained by dominant ideologies and other professional hegemonies. Burke and Harrison conclude that a homeless black single parent could easily be seen as 'undeserving' in struggling to care for his or her child against a background of structural inequalities and racism. This analysis echoes that of Parton et al. (1997) who examine the way in which notions of good enough parenting are constructed and maintained. Ahmad (1993) similarly links the disadvantageous health status of people from black and minority ethnic groups to a wider struggle for equality and against racism. He compares this anti-racist stance to a 'culturist' approach, where realities are constructed and inequalities are explained in terms of cultural differences and deficits, and are addressed not by changes in power relationships but by integration and ethnic sensitivity (Devore and Schlesinger, 1991).

The National Institute for Mental Health in England (NIMHE, 2003) produced a report on improving mental health services for black and minority ethnic communities by a combination of changing service experience and outcome, developing the workforce and engaging the community to develop capacity. Mental health needs are seen as located in a social and cultural context, but also within institutional racism, leading to more frequent use of the Mental Health Act and the criminal justice system for minority ethnic groups. The Sainsbury Centre for Mental Health is presently compiling a national directory of services which work with African and Caribbean communities, following its 2002 report, which showed that lack of information was a major barrier for service users and carers to accessing services before they reach crisis. One recommendation of the report was that 'gateway' organisations should build bridges between the community and services, in order to increase access.

Oppression that is rooted in institutional structures and organisational procedures is harder to penetrate because it is woven into the taken-for-granted life of the agency, and can cover any or all forms of oppression based on status, gender, age or race. It is the outcome or effect of policies or actions that is important, not the intention behind them. This means that different stakeholders – managers, workers and service users – may experience the organisation differently. The tensions between these different experiences were explored in the Macpherson Report (1999), which examined the allegations of racism within the Metropolitan Police and their impact on its investigation into the murder of the black youth, Stephen Lawrence. The report's definition of institutional racism has become generally accepted in emphasising the effects of behaviour rather than the intention (para. 6.34):

> The collective failure of an organisation to provide an appropriate and professional service to people because of their colour, culture and ethnic origin. It can be seen or detected in processes, attitudes and behaviour which amount to discrimination through unwitting prejudice, ignorance, thoughtlessness and racist stereotyping which disadvantage minority ethnic people.

The Macpherson Report accordingly gives the right to define an incident as racist, whether it amounts to a crime or not, predominantly to the victim.

Change at a structural level has been facilitated by the introduction of the Race Relations (Amendment) Act 2000 which places a positive duty on public authorities of all types not to discriminate on the grounds of race, colour, nationality or ethnic or national origin. It covers both direct discrimination or less favourable treatment on racial grounds, and indirect discrimination where a rule is applied to everyone, but can be applied to a smaller proportion of people from particular racial groups for reasons which cannot be justified. The Act also outlaws victimisation of people who have made a complaint of racial discrimination or have supported someone else to do so. The provisions of the Act are also proactive rather than simply reactive, because it also contains a general duty on public authorities, backed up by specific duties, to promote race equality. So, in all of their actions, policies and procedures, public authorities, such as the police, social services, health and education and the justice and welfare systems, must 'mainstream' race equality by having regard to the need to eliminate unlawful discrimination, promote equality and opportunities and promote good race relations.

Disability rights

Thomas (2002) examines the theoretical basis of disability studies from a number of different perspectives, illustrating the different ways in which the experience of disabled people can be understood. Using Thomas's perspectives as a framework, it is possible to point to the following five ways in which practice might be changed, or reframed, in order to practice in an anti-oppressive way.

Materialistic perspectives

Because in capitalist societies, people with disabilities are seen as non-productive in the workforce, the practice response needs to challenge disablist assumptions concerning accessibility and competence. Discrimination as less favourable treatment or a failure to make reasonable adjustments to the working environment to make employment more accessible is unlawful under the Disability Discrimination Act 1996.

Cultural perspectives

Cultural ideas about impairment are founded on the 'binary logic' of 'normativism' versus 'disability' (Derrida, 1998). Cultural ideas about impairment engender disability by setting barriers which locate individuals and groups in positions of powerlessness and dependency. Postmodernism, which challenges the idea of a single or unified identity, emphasises the creativity of social interactions with others which recognises difference as a transformative strength. There is an important cultural challenge here in care/assistance relationships in enabling touch to convey support, whilst forestalling the anxiety evoked by proximity (Price and Shildrick, 2002).

The importance of language in constructing cultural reality and advocating social change is explored by Aspsis (2002). Significant omissions found in 'accessible' information packs on independent living are: information about why people are labelled as 'learning disabled'; definitions of oppression; an analysis of the power of statutory and service agencies; and an explanation of the distinction between ideal and real rights in a legalistic framework. Those presenting information need to take account of these issues properly to achieve their goal of greater choice and increased participation and involvement in the planning of community care (Aspsis, 2002, p. 173).

Phenomenology

The lived experiences of impairment – the social construction of the body as well as disabling barriers – are constructed by social practice; how people actually behave. Judith Butler (1993) calls this 'performativity'; it enables people to experience a range of identities, not solely a disabled identity. This is important, given that oppression frequently works through closing down difference and choice (Corker and Shakespeare, 2002). Giving opportunities for performativity in different social roles, which recognise the diversity of disabled people's lives in terms of gender, race and sexuality, is therefore an important part of anti-oppressive practice.

Psycho-emotional dimensions of disability

Disablist practices that undermine the psychological and emotional well-being of individuals link structured oppression to individual experience in the creation and maintenance of identity. Avery (2002, p. 122) explores the 'identity reconstruction' that parents of children with disabilities face in terms of stigma, and the challenge to core cultural values in 'securing one's child where society sees a patient'. She explains how through the use of internet-linked groups, it is possible to move on from personal tragedy or biomedical discourses on disability to enable parents to reframe their own experience and that of their child. Children also can reject labelling and develop a positive identity through writing, music and play (Peters, 1998).

Human rights

Morris (1994) sees the provision of physical care for people with disabilities as a fundamental human and civil rights issue. Oliver (1996, p. 24) cites the *Fundamental Principles Document of the Union of Physically Impaired against Segregation* which is to seek:

> necessary financial ... and other help required from the State to enable us to gain the maximum possible independence in daily living activities, to achieve mobility, undertake productive work and to live where and how we choose with full control over our own lives.

Matters such as direct payments, adaptations and appropriate housing thus become matters of right rather than negotiation. So Bewley and Glendinning (1994) and Priestley (2003) observed conflicts between disabled people's own definition of independence and those of the statutory authorities. Finkelstein (1993) and Oliver (1996) conclude that insofar as ideas of control and 'needs' rather than rights are at the centre of community care provision, they are almost certain to guarantee the failure of those policies as far as disabled people are concerned.

Mental health and mental capacity

Stigma and discrimination against people with mental health problems has been the subject of a scoping review by NIMHE (2004). The study includes 'expert by experience' evidence, which describes the lived experience of people with mental health problems, and impact assessments, which appraise the effect of public awareness and education programmes and interventions. It was found that the impact of an educational message delivered by a service user is greater than any other form of delivery such as lectures or role play (Pinfold et al., 2003). Translating changing attitudes into changes in behaviour is, however, acknowledged to be more difficult, requiring changes in policy and legislation (such as the Disability Discrimination Act) but, more importantly, community support for change through the inclusion of mental health service users in the workplace and increased opportunities for social contact. Wilson and Beresford (2000) note the failure so far to involve service users significantly in the development of anti-oppressive theory and practice. For student social workers, the issue is that anti-oppressive practice may be seen as a skill to be learned, rather than a political value to be lived. Social work itself, by categorising people as disabled, old or mentally ill, can contribute to this oppression. Much of the social work literature is also taken from an 'expert' perspective, often based on a medical model, whilst research looks at service users as subjects rather than active participants. Thus, the learning and practice of social work itself is to be evaluated according to anti-oppressive principles, with the awareness that it may not be adequate to the task.

In the situation of people who are, or are becoming, mentally incapacitated, that is, unable to make decisions for themselves, the application of values in practice poses real dilemmas for social workers, as this is an area where legislation and professional practice are less well developed. It is an issue which affects people with learning difficulties or mental health problems including dementia. Structural factors such as ageism and racism may be equally relevant to an assessment of the issues. Alhough services such as home care, daycare and respite care can be helpful in delaying the onset of residential care for people with dementia, it is the severity of the person's cognitive impairment which is the most important determining factor for length of stay in the community following referral for social work involvement (Askham and Thompson, 1990; Bland, 1996; Moriarty and Webb, 1997). Services for people from black and ethnic minority communities are definitely underdeveloped, particularly where there is not a large black population (SSI, 1998).

The issue of how directly to involve people with dementia in the planning of their care has not yet been tackled at a strategic level (SSI, 1995a). Goldsmith, (1996) however, is positive that communication with people with dementia is not only possible but necessary for informed decision-making to take place. Knowledge of that person's previous way of life, preferences and personal strengths is essential to predict how well they might adapt to daycare or even what type of residential care they would find amenable. Communication, moreover, need not be only verbal, it can be by gesture or conduct (Dawson and McDonald, 2000; Allen, 2001). As Winner (1992) suggests, this is more than the 'passive consent' that Marsh and Fisher (1992) refer to as the limits of partnership with people with dementia; it is a positive attempt to seek out wishes and feelings.

The 2004 Mental Incapacity Act contains a functional definition of mental incapacity as an inability to comprehend information relevant to a decision, an inability to remember that information and cognitive restrictions on giving weight to different pieces of information to arrive at a choice. The introduction of legislation will clarify the position for both formal and informal carers who provide everyday support such as shopping, cleaning and personal care to people whose mental capacity is in doubt. It will also provide a framework for decision-making by professionals faced with life-changing decisions such as the withdrawal of medical treatment or entry into residential care. Although the BMA has provided guidance for doctors on consent and living wills covering a range of circumstances, and the BMA and Law Society (2003) have produced joint guidance on financial matters, social workers have been relatively unsupported in matters of substitute decision-making (Dawson and McDonald, 2000). As it is unlikely that the power to apply to a reconstructed court of protection for directions on welfare as well as financial matters will be used in any but the most complex cases, agency policies and procedures will need to be developed that are supportive of the key principles contained in the Act. These are:

- There is a presumption of capacity
- Individuals must be supported to make their own decisions, as far as it is practicable to do so
- People are not to be treated as lacking capacity simply because they make unwise decisions
- Everything done for a person lacking capacity is to be done in that person's best interests
- The 'least restrictive option' principle must always be considered.

Assessing capacity

Capacity is a legal concept, although based on evidence of cognitive abilities in respect of the use and retention of information so as to make decisions (or more often, choices) about options available. In a social care context, this may involve consenting to quite a complex package of care. Capacity is not a global concept, but covers a range of issues and the test of capacity for each is different (McDonald and Taylor, 1994), for example the capacity to marry, make a will or enter into a contract. The matter is complicated by the imposition of financial assessments; as Langan and Means (1996) discovered in their research, few local authorities have comprehensive and integrated systems to link financial assessments with delegated financial decision-making through the use of powers of attorney or receivership.

It is important that the assessment of mental capacity precedes substitute decision-making. To this end, it is important to gather sufficient information about the behaviour that is causing concern, but also to set it in the context of other life events such as bereavement or physical ill-health which may affect cognitive functioning. A culturally sensitive assessment will take into account both past history and present needs and will also be relevant to how current behaviour is interpreted. Advocacy services may need to be engaged to support people who find it difficult to speak for themselves.

This is an area replete with professional dilemmas. Social workers need to explore:

- Their own value system and feelings about self-determination and protection from harm
- Legal and ethical boundaries around voluntary and compulsory intervention
- Structural issues relevant to the needs of marginalised groups, such as older people and people with learning difficulties in diverse communities, and the agency's response to those needs
- Fairness in the allocation of resources, if these are limited
- Skill in ascertaining the wishes and feelings of people whose capacity to make decisions needs to be supported
- The rights and feelings of carers.

Frequently, the issues crystallise around support in the community or admission to residential care. In the case of people with dementia, research by Levin et al. (1989) found differences of perception between social workers and carers on the function of daycare and respite care. In some instances, carers saw such services as precursors of permanent residential care, whereas social workers saw such services as a means of keeping people in the community for longer. Such perceptions need to be clarified at the outset. As McPherson (1988) points out, for many older people with dementia, entry into residential care is unregulated, often achieved by stealth and is usually for life, compared to the legal and procedural safeguards which surround admission to a psychiatric hospital. People with dementia may resist the idea of admission to residential care and this may be supported by an analysis of their past views on the subject. Fisher (1990) considers that if there is no mandate from the client, a legal mandate for compulsory intervention must be sought from elsewhere. This could be guardianship under the Mental Health Act, as part of an agreed care plan, or it could be a 'best interests' decision, when it is clear that mental capacity has been lost and the social worker needs to move on from upholding self-determination as the greater good. Yet the emotional cost of a move to residential care would have to be weighed against the physical security that it would provide. Increasing support services in the community might support the family in any decision to withdraw, and would enable the older person with dementia to remain at home until he or she acknowledged that he/she could no longer cope, but the amount of resources needed to achieve this would be very high. The complexity of interlocking values in community care should not therefore be underestimated. Any case is likely to involve the whole gamut from individual to collectivist approaches.

Concluding comments

The specification of social work values has been a contested area. Historically, it has moved beyond the individualist focus of 'respect for persons' to a critical challenge to structural inequalities. Anti-oppressive practice requires a theoretical understanding of the sources of disadvantage and exclusion. Although this chapter concentrated on issues relating to race and disability, it is acknowledged that there is no hierarchy of discriminations and that individuals and groups may suffer multiple disadvantages. Social work practice needs to be sensitive to these multiple identities. The commodification of care that has been associated with community care policies needs to be exposed in order to be challenged. Ways in which it may be challenged include not only the development of advocacy services but also the participation and empowerment of service users in determining policy and contributing to the development of anti-oppressive practice through education and evaluation.

PAUSE AND REFLECT

Find out if policy statements exist locally concerning services for people from black and ethnic groups. Find and describe examples of those services. Do they reflect the values of the communities they serve? How are they publicised? How are they funded?

CASE STUDY

Capacity

Eva Smith, an African-Caribbean woman of 76, lives alone in a three-bedroomed council house. Her husband died two years ago. Her daughters, who visit daily, are concerned that she has become increasingly forgetful, and neighbours have told them that she is in the street late at night, going to the post office 'to collect her pension'. Her daughters approach the social services department saying that they want to talk about residential care for their mother.

How should the allocated worker react?

FURTHER READING

Banks, S. (2001) *Ethics, Accountability and the Social Professions* (2nd edn). Basingstoke: Palgrave – now Palgrave Macmillan.
Explores the origins and development of social work values and compares them to those of related professions.

Dominelli, L. (2002) *Anti-oppressive Social Work – Theory and Practice*. Basingstoke: Palgrave Macmillan.
Links issues of individual human rights to structural disadvantages and discusses the dynamic nature of social work values.

CHAPTER 9

Financial Matters

Introduction

Social workers find that combining a helping relationship with the provision of services subject to a financial assessment is one of the most complex areas of practice (Bradley and Manthorpe, 2000). Yet funding allocations are based on the premise that charges will be made. This chapter looks at the complex rules around paying for community services and residential care. National guidance on charging policies now seeks to limit differences between authorities on ways in which charges are assessed, but also makes it clear that it is part of the assessor's role to maximise the user's income by giving advice on welfare benefits. A brief introduction to welfare benefits is therefore included in this chapter. Service users may also need assistance in planning for the longer term management of their finances, particularly if they are becoming unable to deal with their own affairs. Advising people on the proper use of powers of attorney and receivership as tools for delegated decision-making will be a significant part of the social worker's task, particularly with older people. High on the social policy agenda is the extension of direct payment schemes; as more service users accept direct payments, the role of the social worker will change from a service broker to an enabler. This in itself will test their commitment and that of their agencies to the empowerment of service users.

Social work and financial matters

Social workers have traditionally shown little interest in thinking about financial matters except, perhaps, welfare benefits. The cost of care has been a concern of planners and senior managers, but not individual practitioners. Community care has changed all this. The introduction of a market for care services has meant that services, even the social worker's own time, have to be costed and assessed for value for money. Choice between different options in a care package may be influenced by cost as well as by other qualitative differences between services.

Charging for residential care has always been a requirement of local authorities, imposed by the National Assistance Act 1948, and has always been means-tested for both income and capital. Charging for other services has been discretionary and, apart from meals and transport, historically not widespread (Chetwynd and

Ritchie, 1996). Charging has now, however, become the norm, with the service user cast in the role of consumer. This has implications in a number of ways:

- it may affect assessment practices by introducing affordability issues into a needs-led process
- it focuses attention on the efficiency and effectiveness of services
- it raises administrative issues around charging procedures, the payment of independent providers and recovery of debts.

All this may have to take place within a therapeutic relationship or one which is involuntary. Social workers and their managers also need to be aware of the waning of affect caused by poverty being such a common part of the everyday work of a social services office or voluntary agency. The danger is then that the impact of poverty can be overlooked, ignored or treated superficially (Dowling, 1998).

Charging for services

Local authority charging policies must operate within the law and within guidance. Section 17 of the Health and Social Services and Social Security Adjudications Act 1983 states that charges must be 'reasonable'. Charges must be based only on the income and capital of the service user and not, for example, on that of another member of the household, including a partner or spouse. There should also be a reviewing system to deal with individual challenges to the charges imposed and local authorities should also monitor the effect of changes in charging policy on service take-up and use. A survey by Baldwin and Lunt (1996) into charging policies in six different local authorities found unease and lack of knowledge amongst social workers and wide variations in policy and practice. Many different schemes are possible, based on flat-rate charges, banding, simple and complex means-testing, and single-service or care package assessments. Research by the Disability Alliance casts doubt on the ability of service users to act as real consumers in a mixed economy of care – matching services to costs and making choices (Chetwynd and Ritchie, 1996). Lack of information about how charges were calculated and how they related to the services to be received made it difficult for people to make informed choices about the care they could afford or check if the correct charge had been levied. There was little evidence that people knew that charges were discretionary, that local authorities had the power to waive charges or were required to continue statutory services, even though charges were not paid. Looking at where the money comes from to be able to afford care raises the whole question of the purpose of disability benefits. If disability benefits such as disability living allowance and attendance allowance are supports for independent living, to impose charges based on this income is to impose a penalty for disability.

In a survey of disabled service users, Rummery (2002) found that people were unhappy about paying for inflexible services delivered at inconvenient times. Nor did paying for services enable people to exit the system, in the absence of a well-developed market for social care. For some people, paying service charges appeared to act as a barrier to citizenship by increasing poverty and thus social isolation and marginalisation. For others, paying family and friends to undertake tasks for them was seen not in terms of consumerism, but in terms of social reciprocity and competence. This is an important finding because it acts as a warning that the 'commodification' of care may undermine reciprocal social relationships, if formal services are inadequate or have been refused.

How should social workers respond to these dilemmas within charging systems? Chetwynd and Ritchie (1996) found that assessments were perceived by users to have worked best when there was honesty and a high degree of interaction between the service user and assessor. Users should also be informed of their rights in order to challenge assessments seen to be unreasonable. The importance of regular review and making users aware of how and in what circumstances they may apply for more help is emphasised in the research as an assurance that users with fluctuating needs will not be overlooked.

The standardisation of charging policies was a late development in community care. Bradley and Manthorpe (2000) found that charging regimes continued to vary widely and social workers continued to be confused and unhappy with their implementation. Current guidance (DoH, 2001i) now sets out for the first time a national framework designed to ensure that charging policies are fair and operate consistently. Nothing in the guidance requires councils to make pre-existing charging policies less generous to service users, indeed, they may choose to levy no charges at all. The guidance, however, lays down the following principles that seek to address some of the difficulties disclosed in the research:

- Users receiving income support or income-based jobseeker's allowance, with a 25 per cent 'buffer', will not be charged for services
- Users in receipt of disability living allowance, attendance allowance or severe disability premium should have an individual assessment of their disability-related expenditure
- Earnings should be disregarded as part of income
- Local authorities should provide benefits advice to enable people to maximise their income.

The obligation to provide benefits advice clarifies the responsibilities of social workers in the area of welfare rights, and the requirement to conduct disability assessments should ensure that the true costs of disability are taken into account. Most importantly, for the first time, there has been an attempt to implement distributive justice by setting principles for charging on a national basis.

Direct payments

The emphasis in legislation historically has been on local authority provision of services, and a prohibition (reiterated in the *Policy Guidance* – DoH, 1990) on cash payments instead of services. This has limited choice and not enabled service users to act as their own care managers in a way seen as empowering by Smale and Tuson (1993).

The Community Care (Direct Payments) Act 1996 came into force in April 1997. The Act gave SSDs the power to make direct cash payments to individuals in lieu of the community care services they have assessed those individuals as needing. Legislative changes introduced by the Health and Social Care Act 2001, sections 57 and 58, have effectively imposed a duty rather than a power on local authorities to make direct payments to any adult who is eligible and would benefit from direct payments, including those over 65, and to disabled 16–17-year-olds (introduced under the Carers and Disabled Children Act 2000). Also, performance indicators will require local authorities to show that direct payments have been discussed as an option with service users, rather than leaving this choice to the discretion of assessors. The regulations which prevented services from being provided by close relatives have also been relaxed. It is now possible (Community Care, Services for Carers and Children (Direct Payments) (England) Regulations 2003) to secure services from a close relative living in the same household, if it is 'necessary to meet satisfactorily the prescribed person's need for that service', or (in the case of Children Act services) 'necessary for promoting the welfare of a child in need'. However, the local authority may require that the payee does not secure a relevant service from a particular individual. Thus, the two separate streams of social policy – direct payments and support for carers – which had been allowed to develop without any real reference to each other are, in this context, being brought more closely together.

Direct payments will not replace care provided by the NHS, cover housing costs or fund long-term residential care. The direct payments scheme is itself subject to existing policy and practice guidance on community care generally but specific guidance was updated in the light of legislative changes (DoH, 2003c). However, it is up to individual authorities to decide how flexible their own schemes should be, how often payments should be made and for what services. All direct payments should, however, form part of a care plan and should follow on from a comprehensive assessment. The legislative framework requires that:

- The person for whom the direct payment is made must be 'willing and able' to manage the direct payments and retain overall control over the money and the final responsibility for how much is spent. This should be monitored and reviewed. Repayment for mismanagement of funds may be required
- Any financial contributions due from the user will be taken into account in setting the amount of direct payment
- The local authority has a duty to step in as backup in emergencies to meet assessed needs.

In principle, direct payments seem to offer an alternative opportunity for users to prioritise their own spending on care services and choose their own providers. Local authorities should not set a condition that only certain providers should be used. Monitoring of quality is thus, initially at least, the user's own responsibility and choice (Dawson, 2000). Hasler and Stewart (2004) highlight the importance of champions in showing local authorities how direct payments can help to increase user involvement and support independent living. Direct payments schemes appear to be most successful when local authorities fund user-led support services as part of their mainstream provision.

Already the number of people with physical disabilities receiving direct payments has shown an increase of 27 per cent in the year 2002–3, rising from

4,274 to 5,459 (SSI, 2003). However, although the number of older people receiving direct payments almost doubled in the same period, total figures were a modest 1,032, and the potential of direct payments for reducing stigma and social exclusion and promoting independence and rehabilitation among people with mental health problems 'is simply not being exploited' (SSI, 2003). In his survey of users of direct payments, Stainton (2002) found them overwhelmingly positive about direct payments, often speaking in emancipatory language. Significantly, users' experiences did not bear out workers' fears of problems in finding staff, risk and health and safety issues. Research into the receipt of direct payments specifically by older people (Clark et al., 2004) and people with learning difficulties (Holman, 2000) similarly showed the importance of positive attitudes within agencies and by workers to extend the use of direct payments. Support and payroll services, advocacy and the use of user-controlled trusts are all means of increasing the accessibility of direct payments to people who need assistance to manage. In particular, support for people with communication difficulties is important so that the presumption in favour of their capacity to consent to direct payments can be given effect to. Similarly, the ability of direct payments to promote independence for people with learning difficulties is congruent with *Valuing People* (DoH, 2000b), and rigid interpretations of 'willing and able' should not be used to constrain eligibility (Dawson and McDonald, 2000).

Before 1993, additional cash payments for severely disabled people were available from the independent living fund supported by monies from central government. After 1993, this money was replaced by the independent living (continuation) fund for existing claimants, and the independent living fund for new claimants. Preference is given to younger disabled people seeking to live independently. The minimum financial support given is for care in excess of a £275 floor provided by the social services authority. Any need for care above the value of £500 per week reverts to the local authority. Money is paid directly to the disabled person. Only persons under the age of 65 are eligible. For younger people with disabilities, a complex package of care can be put together, using direct payments in tandem with money from the independent living fund, although access to both is still gained by a community care assessment.

Welfare benefits

Being aware of the range and type of benefits available is a necessary part of effective working in community care. Maximising income enables people to buy in resources not otherwise available and exercise choice. For this reason, some welfare rights services concentrate on take-up campaigns rather than advice in individual cases.

Benefits may be either contributory or non-contributory, that is, dependent on a minimum number of NI contributions having been paid or available regardless of contribution record. Non-contributory benefits can be means-tested or non-means-tested. Income replacement benefits such as income support are means-tested and are payable only below a certain threshold of need. Other benefits, such as disability living allowance, are compensatory benefits and are based on eligibility criteria which are independent of income. Payment of benefit may be affected by stays in residential care, hospital or prison, for which different rules apply.

Some benefits are highly specialised, such as war pensions and industrial injuries benefits, and will not be dealt with here. What follows is an outline of the major income replacement and disability benefits available. An important recent trend has been the introduction of tax credits to replace welfare benefits. This is part of the government's welfare-to-work programme, given effect to by the New Deal. The DWP now deals with social security benefits, but tax credits are dealt with by the Inland Revenue. Social exclusion is to be tackled through a greater emphasis on opportunity to join the workforce, for example for young people and single parents, rather than the unrestricted availability of benefits.

Jobseeker's allowance

Jobseeker's allowance applies to all those who are required to 'sign on' as available for work as a condition of receiving benefit. There are two types of jobseeker's allowance: contribution-based (which lasts for six months and is paid independently of other income) and income-based (which is means-tested). Claimants are required to sign a jobseeker's agreement and agree to their 'pattern of availability', which is normally being available for work up to 40 hours each week. The eligibility criteria for jobseeker's allowance are stringent, and after six months claimants can be required to take work which is different from, and less well paid than, the work they are used to doing. Those with caring responsibilities may however limit their hours of availability to fewer than the normal minimum of 24 hours per week. People who have a disability, physical or mental, but who are not eligible for incapacity benefit (see below) may limit the type of work they are able to do without having to show that they have still a reasonable prospect of securing employment.

Income support

Income support is available as an income maintenance benefit for those who are not required to sign on for work, for example those with dependent children. It can also be a top-up to other benefits. Payment of income support is based on a formula whereby the 'applicable amount' (the amount deemed necessary to live on) minus any income from other sources is the amount of income support to be paid. The applicable amount comprises a personal allowance plus any premiums to which the claimant is entitled. There are premiums for disability and carers.

Tax credits

The move away from means-tested benefits to tax credits has had a major impact on income support. Child tax credit (CTC) and working tax credit (WTC) were introduced in April 2003 and are administered not as part of the benefits system, but by the Inland Revenue. In the case of a couple, the award may be split between the one who is in work (WTC) and the carer of the child (CTC). For

WTC, the claimant must be at least 16 and work at least 16 hours a week. There is a separate category for claimants aged at least 25 and working at least 30 hours as week, as well as for those over 50 coming off benefits and into work and for people with a disability. Up to 70 per cent of authorised childcare costs are taken into account. Child benefit remains as a separate universal non-means-tested benefit. For pensioners, the minimum income guarantee, which was effectively an income support top-up for the state pension, is replaced by pension credit which has a more generous threshold and gives credit for modest savings as well as low income.

The social fund

The social fund covers needs arising from exceptional circumstances that cannot be met from normal income. There are both discretionary and non-discretionary payments. Discretionary payments are paid out of a fixed annual budget. Although there is national guidance on priority groups (the elderly, disabled, families under stress) and district priorities (details of which should be publicly available), each case should be treated on its merits. For unsuccessful claimants, there is a two-stage review process; an internal local office review and a social fund inspector review. There are three types of discretionary payments: crisis loans, budgeting loans and community care grants.

Anyone can apply for a crisis loan, not just those getting income support. Crisis loans are available for emergencies, being 'the only way that serious damage or serious risk to health or safety can be prevented' (McDonald, 2004). Living expenses at the beginning of benefits claims may be paid by way of a crisis loan. Budgeting loans are available only to those continuously on income support for six months or more; the minimum loan is £30. Furniture, bedding, clothing and home repairs are a priority. Such loans are not available for domestic assistance in the home. Deposits to secure accommodation are not covered, but rent in advance to secure board and lodging or hostel accommodation is possible.

Community care grants are intended to cover:

- re-establishment in the community following a period in institutional or residential care (usually of three months or more, but this is not an absolute rule)
- support to remain in the community
- travel in the UK to cover a domestic crisis
- a visit to a sick person
- a move to more suitable accommodation.

Savings of under £500 (£1,000 if aged over 60) are disregarded. It is advisable to cost items sought, for example from a catalogue. The usual items covered are furniture and bedding, clothing, removal expenses, fuel connection charges, laundry needs and travel needs (when a lump sum for up to 26 weeks can be awarded). Community care grants may be claimed not only to allow a disabled person, for example, to move into more suitable accommodation, but also to enable a carer to move to live with a person for whom they will provide care.

Non-discretionary payments are maternity payments, payments for funeral expenses and cold weather payments. The Sure Start maternity payment is a one-off payment of £500. Funeral expenses (up to a maximum of £600) are payable only to the person responsible for arranging the funeral, a test which has become narrower in recent years. Cold weather payments, payable for periods of very cold weather, do not need to be claimed but will be paid automatically to people on means-tested benefits who are pensioners or disabled or who have a child under five. Winter fuel payments, available to all those over 60, are paid independently of the social fund and are not means-tested.

Retirement pensions

Entitlement to a retirement pension depends on the following factors:

- having reached 'pensionable age' (currently 65 for a man and 60 for a woman)
- making a claim for a pension to be paid
- satisfying contribution conditions.

The pension paid may consist of a basic pension, plus an additional pension (payable under the SERPS scheme unless contracted out) and a graduated pension (based on contributions between April 1961 and April 1975). There is a small age addition for those over 80. The Pensions Service will give individuals a 'pension forecast' on request. All retirement pensions are taken fully into account for tax credit purposes.

Bereavement benefits

Bereavement benefits are payable to both men and women, under pension age. Benefits depend upon the NI contributions of the person who has died. There is a £2,000 lump sum bereavement payment, a bereavement allowance paid to people aged 45 or over, which is paid for 52 weeks and a widowed parent's allowance for people with dependent children.

Incapacity benefit

Incapacity benefit is payable to people who are unable to work due to sickness or disability and who have paid sufficient NI contributions. Incapacity benefit without a contribution condition has replaced severe disablement allowance for those disabled before the age of 20. There are two tests:

- the 'own occupation' test which applies for the first six months of incapacity
- the 'all work' test which applies thereafter, or from the beginning of a claim if there was no usual occupation.

Incapacity for work is assessed according to a functional test of disability across a range of competences which cover both physical and mental impairments. Some people are deemed to have passed the test of incapacity by virtue of the nature of their condition, others will have to satisfy a DWP doctor that they are incapable of work if their condition is not chronic. The position of people with mental health problems is particularly problematic, as only recognised forms of mental disorder will constitute incapacity. This has the effect of excluding people with minor forms of mental disorder such as anxiety states.

There are difficulties in filling in claim forms allowing only yes/no answers, and problems with medicals which ignore pain, fatigue, variability and length of time taken to complete an activity. Appeals, however, have had a relatively high success rate. Incapacity benefit is paid at short- and long-term rates (long term after 12 months' incapacity), but unlike its predecessor invalidity benefit, it is not payable to people of pensionable age. One million of the 2.4 million claimants of incapacity benefit are aged over 50.

Disability living allowance and attendance allowance

Benefits which are compensatory for disability are payable on the basis of need, regardless of income or capital. Disability living allowance consists of a care component and a mobility component, while attendance allowance is payable to those over the age of 65 and only has a care component. There is no need to show that the benefit is used to purchase care or that care is actually given. Entitlement is based on the effects of disability on a person's life rather than the presence of a particular disabling condition. There are three rates for the care component of disability living allowance – lower, middle and higher – but only two rates of attendance allowance – higher and lower – corresponding to the higher and middle rates of disability living allowance.

The lower rate of the care component of disability living allowance is payable to people aged under 65 who need 'limited attention', for example getting up and going to bed, or people over the age of 16 but under 65 who are unable to prepare a cooked main meal for themselves. Many people with learning disabilities will be eligible for the lower rate. The middle rate of disability living allowance is available to those who need frequent attention (for example help with toileting) or continual supervision throughout the day or night. The higher rate is payable to those who are in need of attention or supervision day and night (most people in residential care will qualify for this). Children may be awarded disability living allowance if their care needs are substantially greater than the needs of other children of the same age.

The mobility component of disability living allowance is payable over the age of three, and, if awarded before the age of 65, it will continue beyond that age. Although the higher and lower rate tests for the mobility component appear to be two halves of a unified benefit, in effect the criteria they employ are so different that they are best considered separately. The higher rate is available to those who are unable, or virtually unable, to walk or who are both deaf and blind and need someone with them when outdoors. The lower rate is payable to those who can walk but who need someone with them when outdoors, or who are severely mentally impaired, with severe behavioural problems. People with cardiovascular complaints who find it difficult to walk any distance out of doors may qualify.

To receive disability living allowance, help must have been needed for three months (six months for attendance allowance). There is a special procedure for people who are terminally ill, that is, not expected to live longer than six months; application may be made by someone other than the recipient who need not then be informed of the prognosis for their condition.

Banks (2003) has carried out research into the impact of disability living allowance in Scotland. Ninety three per cent of respondents said that they found the disability living allowance claim form difficult to complete, some found it upsetting and 80 per cent had to get help to complete it. Delays in decision-making were seen as unacceptable, and the review and renewal process was a significant source of anxiety for most respondents. Worryingly, there was a danger of people being 'penalised for coping', if they brought in help which diminished the need for the benefit. There may be an inhibition about fully describing the extent of one's disability on the form; needing encouragement to take medication or care for oneself should not be overlooked as a basis for a claim. There is obviously an important role for the social worker here in enabling people to appraise honestly the extent of their disability and fit it within the benefits criteria which are described.

Carers allowance

This allowance is paid to the carer, not to the person who is cared for. It is an income replacement benefit with no upper age limit which is payable only to those who provide 'regular and substantial care' to one individual for 35 hours per week or more. Carers allowance is not means-tested, but is taxable and subject to the rules on overlapping benefits and so cannot be paid out at the same time as, for example, bereavement benefit or retirement pension. An underlying entitlement to carers allowance will, however, attract the carers premium included in the calculation of income support, housing benefit and council tax benefit. A major disadvantage in claiming carers allowance is that the person being cared for loses his or her entitlement to the severe disability premium for income support (which is substantial).

Housing benefit

Housing benefit may be available to people on low income who have capital of less than £16,000 to cover the payment of rent, including board and lodging and hostel payments. It will not be paid on rents deemed to be 'unreasonably high' (as determined by the valuation officer) and will only be paid on the 'eligible rent', which will exclude payment for such items as heating and laundry costs. Payments for care or support services are funded by providers through *Supporting People* grants. Housing benefit is not available for those living with close relatives unless payment is on a strictly commercial basis or the accommodation is self-contained (such as a granny flat).

Council tax benefit

Council tax is payable on the basis of one bill per dwelling, regardless of the number of people living there – although a single-person household will automatically receive a 25 per cent discount. A second adult rebate (maximum 25 per cent) is available if a second person with a low income is living with the householder. A 'status discount' also applies to people who are severely mentally impaired – they pay no council tax – and to live-in carers of people in receipt of the higher or middle rate of the care component of disability living allowance or attendance allowance. Disabled people who need additional space for wheelchair use, or a second bathroom, may apply under the disability reduction scheme to have the valuation of their property reduced by one band.

Going into hospital or residential care

Particular rules apply to benefits received by people who are in hospital and after 12 months in hospital only a basic personal allowance will be paid. Dependants of people who are in hospital for more than 12 months may apply to the DWP to be assessed in their own right as single claimants. Entitlement to disability living allowance or attendance allowance is lost after a stay of 28 days in hospital or publicly funded residential care; periods of care separated by less than 28 days are counted together for reasons of eligibility. Periods of respite care should be carefully planned with this in mind. There are indefinite exemptions from council tax for people in hospital or residential care; this exemption also applies to carers who leave their own home to live elsewhere to give personal care. Housing benefit may be paid to cover absences of up to 52 weeks in hospital, but is limited to 13 weeks for people in residential accommodation for a trial period, and for convicted prisoners.

Paying for residential and nursing home care

Local authorities are required to charge for the care that they provide in residential or nursing homes by section 22 of the National Assistance Act 1948; they have no discretion not to do so. The Department of Health regularly publishes guidance and updates on the factors to be taken into account on assessment. Under the Charging for Residential Accommodation Guide (CRAG) rules, residents will be assessed on their income and capital (up to a current maximum of £20,500). There is no legal requirement for a spouse to disclose his or her income and assets; all that the local authority can do is seek an agreement with this person as a 'liable relative', while other relatives have no obligation to contribute to the cost of care. However, a relative may voluntarily enter into a third party agreement to 'top up' the cost of care beyond the local authority's usual maximum. Those people who were funded by the DSS as having 'preserved rights' before 31 March 1993 are now the responsibility of the local authority in which they are ordinarily resident. If accommodation is provided under section 117 of the Mental Health Act 1983, no charge can be made for it, just as no charge can be made for any other community care service thus provided.

Having to sell one's home to meet residential or nursing home fees is a frequent source of contention and 40,000 people annually are in this position. The value of the property is not taken into account for the first three months and is not counted at all when a spouse or partner, a relative over the age of 60 or someone who is disabled remains living there. In other cases, the local authority has a discretion to ignore the value of the property. If the owner does not wish to sell, a legal charge can be placed on the property as part of the resident's estate or a deferred payment agreement can be entered into. The charge then becomes payable to the local authority upon death. Different rules apply to temporary residents. Local authorities may at their discretion impose a reduced or flat-rate charge for short-term care for periods up to eight weeks. The value of property is not taken into account in short-term care assessments or for temporary residents whose stay is unlikely to exceed 52 weeks.

Deprivation of capital in order to reduce the accommodation charge is dealt with under CRAG rules and the Health and Social Services and Social Security Adjudications Act 1983. Although there is no time limit on the tracing back of capital, the CRAG makes it clear that the timing of the disposal should be taken into account when considering the purpose of the disposal. It would be unreasonable to decide that a resident had disposed of an asset in order to reduce his or her charge for accommodation when the disposal took place at a time when he or she was fit and healthy and could not have foreseen the need for a move to residential accommodation. Statistically, the chance of entering residential care (a maximum 1 in 4) is less than the chance of a relative's marriage breaking down or them becoming unemployed and unable to pay a continuing mortgage. Law Society rules require solicitors to clarify in these circumstances who the client is, so that if a conflict of interest arises, the relatives may need to be separately represented (see McDonald and Taylor, 1995).

Paying for long-term care

Discontent at the cost of long-term care and a system which penalised people for saving and acquiring assets over their lifetime (Age Concern, 1994) has led to a review of long-term care policy. The House of Commons Health Committee (1996) considered a number of insurance-based schemes, but acknowledged that people would need a financial incentive to enter into such schemes. The issue is as much a moral and political one as a legal one, and the question is ripe for wider public debate (Diba, 1996). A Royal Commission on Long Term Care was appointed in 1999 to consider both social and financial issues, and by a majority recommended that personal care, wherever located, should be free of charge. This recommendation has been implemented in Scotland, but not in England and Wales. By an Amendment to the National Assistance Act 1948, however, the nursing element of nursing home care can no longer be charged for and eligibility for continuing NHS care has also been clarified (see Chapter 10); however personal (social care), wherever located, is still subject to means-testing.

Financial management

Dealing with the financial affairs of vulnerable adults raises professional dilemmas for the social worker. Bradley and Manthorpe (1995) describe this work as 'beyond welfare rights', insofar as it requires practitioners to monitor expenditure and offer protection to people who may be vulnerable to exploitation. Research by Langan and Means (1994) found responsibility divided between social workers and staff and officers in the finance departments of local authorities. The latter were often critical of social workers for overlooking financial matters. However, the workshops organised by Bradley and Manthorpe confirmed that social workers (working in this instance with older people) welcomed opportunities to discuss problems in the delegation of financial responsibility, feelings about the deprivation of capital and reactions to the possibility of financial abuse by relatives.

A brief account of legal devices for delegating financial responsibility is considered below, but for further details, see Letts (1998) and McDonald and Taylor (1995).

Agency and appointeeship

An agency comes into being when one person (the principal) delegates to another (the agent) responsibility for a given transaction. Commonly, this takes place when another person is authorised to collect a social security benefit for another. However, if the person becomes incapable of handling their own financial affairs, it is possible for that other person to become their appointee; the benefit is then given out in the name of the appointee and the collection of the money and any dealings with the DWP become their responsibility. They are still bound, of course, to use the money for the benefit of the person for whom they act as appointee. Local authorities may act as appointees for the people they place in residential care and although owners of residential homes are discouraged from becoming appointees, in practice this often happens because there is no one else to do the job. Monitoring of this should take place through the biannual inspections of care homes by the CSCI.

Ordinary and enduring powers of attorney

A power of attorney is a formal document made by deed which appoints another person (or persons) to act on behalf of the donor in financial matters. This may be a general power, or it may be limited to particular transactions. The donor does not lose his or her own right to act, but in effect shares it. The difference between an ordinary and enduring power of attorney is that the former is no longer valid if the donor should become mentally incapacitated. However, an enduring power of attorney does remain valid when the donor becomes mentally incapacitated. Enduring powers of attorney have to be registered with the Public Guardianship Office (the executive arm of the court of protection) when incapacity is reached; thereafter they cannot be revoked. Enduring powers of attorney are immensely useful if a trusted friend or relative can manage the financial affairs of someone whose mental capacity is likely to deteriorate. These are overwhelmingly private arrangements; local authorities on the whole do not act as attorneys for their clients (Langan and Means, 1994). The Mental Capacity Act 2004 proposes the introduction of a new lasting power of attorney which will facilitate the delegation not only of financial but also welfare and healthcare decisions.

Receivership

Mental capacity is needed to grant a power of attorney; if this has already been lost, then an application to the Public Guardianship Office for the appointment of a receiver is the only legal avenue. Local authorities may initiate receivership and may be appointed receiver. Annual accounts must be submitted and a fidelity bond is required. The procedure is costly, and those with capital of less than £5,000 are unlikely to come within the jurisdiction. Langan and Means (1994) found that few local authorities had considered the advocacy role of the receiver in securing access to community care services. Indeed, one of the difficulties of the present system is that it separates out the responsibility for financial decisions from responsibility for personal well-being, not only in the area of receipt of services, but also in the decision of where an individual might live and the range of people with whom he or she may come into contact. Thus, for example, a receiver has no authority to negotiate a placement in residential care, although she or he will be expected to finance that placement if one is made.

The social worker's role

Social workers have come in for criticism from the local government ombudsman for failing to provide proper information about welfare benefits. In a complaint against Humberside County Council, delay, amounting to maladministration, in securing 24-hour care for a severely disabled man discharged from hospital had been caused by the social worker's failure to apply for the highest rate of the care component of disability living allowance as a prerequisite for an application to the independent living fund. Similarly, in another case involving East Sussex County Council, a social worker's statement that a person registered as blind was not entitled to additional benefits was inaccurate, and therefore maladministration. In fact the claimant was entitled to severe disablement allowance because of her disability. Interestingly, in this case the ombudsman interpreted the duty placed on local authorities by s.9 of the Disabled Persons Act 1986 to provide information about 'any relevant services' as including the giving of advice about welfare benefits. This places welfare rights advice amongst the statutory duties of local authorities. The need for social workers to be able to assess the financial costs of disability and provide advice on income maximisation is strengthened by the fairer charging policy guidance (DoH, 2000i).

Concluding comments

Social work involvement in legal and financial matters, and the growing need for knowledge and expertise in this field, opens up the possibility of whole new areas of interprofessional working – with advice agencies and lawyers in particular. Both professions have an obligation to clarify in a complex family situation 'who the client is', and act in the best short- and long-term interests of that client. Given the desire of many people to 'put their house in order', the making of a proper will or an enduring power of attorney are matters which may need to be discussed, and could well be the subject of a referral on for independent legal advice. Joint guidance provided by the BMA/Law Society (2003) on assessing mental capacity is also relevant to social workers. At a minimum, social workers will need to have an awareness of basic welfare rights knowledge and local authority financial policies, acknowledging that this is part of the statutory framework in which they work. Research has shown that service users need reliable information about charges and that they value openness and honesty in this respect. They may also require support to pursue claims in a political climate which may stigmatise those in receipt of benefits as 'dependent', and there is evidence that application procedures act as a real barrier to establishing entitlement. There is an absence of informed public debate about the proper boundaries between health and social care, which is of concern, given that healthcare services are free at the point of delivery. Interagency working between health and social care is the subject of Chapter 10.

PAUSE AND REFLECT

Find out details of your local authority scheme for direct payments. Does it cover people with learning disabilities and mental health problems, as well as those with physical disabilities? How does the local authority decide whether a person is 'able' and willing' to receive direct payments instead of services? Is any evaluation being undertaken of the effectiveness of such a scheme?

CASE STUDY

Welfare benefits

Joan Shaw, aged 58, cares for her son James, aged 26, who lives nearby and has mental health problems. James has a diagnosis of bipolar disorder; sometimes he is very low and needs motivating to look after himself and his flat and mix with other people, and at other times he refuses to sleep and has run up large debts after going on spending sprees with strangers. Joan feels that she needs to visit James every day to see how he is managing. Joan has a morning cleaning job for which she earns £50 per week. James has recently had to give up his job as a computer programmer because he was unable to concentrate and his ability to attend work was erratic.

What benefits and support may Joan and James be entitled to?

FURTHER READING

Bateman, N. (2000) *Advocacy Skills for Health and Social Care Professionals*. London: Jessica Kingsley.
A practical guide to advocacy and representation, including appeals advocacy within the social security system.

Bradley, G. and Manthorpe, J. (1997) *Dilemmas of Financial Assessment: A Practitioner's Guide.* Birmingham: Venture Press.
Explores and explains the real-life dilemmas that social workers face in carrying out financial assessments and the variety of organisational arrangements that exist to support vulnerable adults who are unable to manage their own financial affairs.

Richards, M. (2001) *Long-term Care for Older People: Law and Financial Planning.* Bristol: Jordan. Written by a lawyer, explains the financial implications of entering long-term care.

CHAPTER 10

Social and Healthcare Needs

Introduction

The universalism of healthcare means that everyone has an interest in health policy and practice. Many service users also have specific healthcare needs as well as social care needs and interagency working is fundamental to the effective delivery of a cohesive package of care. There have been significant developments since 1999 towards a primary care-led NHS. At the same time, performance indicators have emphasised the importance of throughput and thus have prioritised acute care. The implication of these trends for joint working is discussed in the light of new legislation and guidance, within systems which are increasingly being combined through the use of section 31 Health Act 1999 flexibilities. This chapter looks at problems in the definition of social care and healthcare needs, the development of the NHS outside local government and three areas which illustrate points of contact between systems: hospital discharge, continuing care and mental health services.

Definitions of healthcare and social care

There is no firmly fixed boundary between what is healthcare and what is social care. Government guidance is notable by its absence in this area, which means that individual health authorities and social services agencies have to work together to produce local guidance on where the boundaries lie between different services (Banks, 2002). The legal responsibility of the NHS is still 'to provide a comprehensive healthcare service designed to secure improvement in the physical and mental health of the nation' (National Health Service Act 1977, s.1), and the Health Act 1999 in section 27 includes a statutory duty to cooperate.

The reason why coordination between health and social care is so difficult to achieve in practice often relates back to historical divergences between services, compounded by different budgetary arrangements and, in some cases, by a difference in perspectives between services or between individuals within them (Glasby and Littlechild, 2004). The role of healthcare services in promoting well-being is controversial. The relationship between poor health and poverty is well known; healthcare services may not be uniformly available to all sections of the population. There are geographical variations in the availability of services according to local priorities, and the priority normally given to acute care cases may mean cutbacks in services for people with chronic conditions, particularly older people and those with long-term mental illness. Personal responsibility for health is emphasised in prevention strategies covering issues such as smoking, obesity and sexual health.

Overlapping responsibilities and anomalies may arise; for example Age Concern (1994) drew attention to risible definitions of what constitutes a social bath (responsibility of social services) and what constitutes a medical bath (responsibility of the health authority). Now that the home help service has become largely a home care service, the point at which the responsibilities of the home care assistant end and that of, say, a community nurse begin will need definition. Although dressing wounds and giving intravenous injections are clearly nursing activities, there are often areas of overlap, where local agreements may have decided that an individual home care assistant may, for example, give injections to an individual patient who is diabetic.

Changes in the NHS

The 1990s saw the introduction of the internal market within the NHS which built in a split between purchasers and providers and saw competition as the way in which efficiency between different providers could be increased (DoH, 1989). With notions of competition being replaced by those of partnership (Balloch and Taylor, 2001), the formal internal market has been dismantled but a commissioning role remains with PCTs and a providing role continues to be performed by NHS trusts. Success in the providing role is to be rewarded with greater independence from central control by the introduction of foundation hospital status. Quality in healthcare services is assured through the operation of clinical governance principles and a focused accountability to strategic health authorities. The Modernisation Agency within the Department of Health is the central means of pushing forward internal reform. Joint investment plans (JIPs) are used to coordinate services between health and other agencies. Section 31 of the Health Act 1999 introduced flexibilities, enabling the pooling of budgets and lead commissioning to be introduced as well as the sharing of personnel and resources to carry out statutory functions, leading to opportunities for joint professional teams in adult services. The development of health services in the latter part of the 1990s and beyond has been driven by a number of factors:

- The opportunity for a more seamless service with social care
- A greater emphasis on accountability for meeting targets and key performance indicators as quality measures
- A drive towards more patient and carer involvement through formal systems
- A primary care-led NHS, with PCTs controlling 75 per cent of the total NHS budget and GPs being given more freedom of choice about working conditions and patient care.

So how has this come about?

Managerialism

Managerialism and competition within the internal market of the NHS has had several consequences for patients at the level of primary and secondary care. At the level of primary care, the new GPs' contract of 1990 introduced the principle of open lists, meaning that patients may move freely now from one GP practice to another; conversely, GPs may remove patients whom they deem to be unsuitable from their lists. This newly created competition between GP practices, combined with opportunities for fundholders to manage their own costs, led to what Holliday (1995) calls 'skimming' and 'skimping'. 'Skimming' is the process of shedding patients who make greater than average demands on practice budgets or GPs' time. 'Skimping' is the rationing of resources by cautious prescribing of medications or selective referral to secondary services (New and LeGrand, 1996). Initiatives such as the Patients Charter also gave a premium to acute care and rapid response in preference to services with strong social components requiring expensive and long-term involvement. The radical agenda advocated by the Black Report continued to be ignored (Townsend and Davidson, 1992). Looking at the disparities in health status (both mental and physical health) between different income groups, the Black Report (DHSS, 1980) recommended a broad programme of public action covering not only health but also unemployment and housing. Although there is now an emphasis on preventive healthcare, the approach is largely based on personal responsibility for health; an approach reiterated in the White Paper on public health (DoH, 2004c).

The responsibilities of the NHS Executive have been passed to regional directors of health and social care and old style health authorities have been replaced by 28 strategic health authorities, covering larger areas. Provisions in the Health and Social Care Act 2001 to enable PCTs or NHS trusts to combine with local authorities to be designated as 'care trusts' have not, however, been much used. Greater use has been made of the section 31 flexibilities in the Health Act 1999 for pooling budgets and joint commissioning. An integrated care pathway approach is also increasingly being used as a means of agreeing local referral and treatment protocols between agencies. 'Partnership' trusts, especially in mental health, have developed for the exchange of statutory functions. Overview and scrutiny committees established under the Local Government Act 2000 have had their role extended to provide a democratic review of health service functions and, in particular, any plans for a 'substantial variation' in health provision locally. Patient-focused benchmarking has also been introduced for healthcare practitioners (DoH, 2001f).

Openness and accountability

The impetus towards openness and accountability within the NHS was increased following the report into the death of children in Bristol following heart surgery (DoH, 2002). The old system of community health councils has been abolished in England (but not in Wales). The Commission for Patient and Public Involvement in Health has been created to act as a bridge between the newly created patients forums and government. In addition to being monitoring bodies for every PCT and NHS trust in England, patients forums will also provide independent advice and information on the making of complaints by individual patients. The internal regulation of quality and performance monitoring in the NHS is carried out through a system of clinical governance and is inspected by CHAI. Additionally, NICE advises the NHS on treatment options and prescribing. The modernisation agenda will also be driven forward by a Modernisation Agency, Leadership Centre and University of the NHS (DoH, 2001). At an individual practitioner level, the regulatory powers of the existing professional bodies are to be overseen by a new Council for the Regulation of Healthcare Professionals. The terms of service of GPs have also changed with the introduction of a new GMS contract, which enables GPs to manage their personal workload according to their interests and patients needs and offer so-called 'enhanced' services, such as minor surgery, that cross the boundary between secondary and primary care.

Service developments

The traditional dualism between primary and secondary care has been joined by a third type of care, intermediate care (particularly for older people). Intermediate care has been developed, using existing as well as new resources, for those people who would otherwise be admitted inappropriately to hospital or have their discharge delayed (DoH, 2002e). Joint planning between health and social care is again emphasised and this is supported by the introduction of JIPs for older people's services, mental health and learning disability. In addition, £300 million was allocated to local authorities for the period 2001–03 through the building care capacity grant to foster agreement between the statutory and independent social care, healthcare and housing sectors, while private finance initiatives enable private sector funding to be brought in. The mixed economy of care thus continues to be fostered in order to meet demands for service. Significant in the development of national standards has been the introduction of NSFs, most notably those for older people and mental health. Although health-led, the frameworks also impose targets on social care through the setting of standards for service design and delivery.

Partnership working

The shift from a contract culture to one of partnership in the delivery of health and social care is exemplified in *Shifting the Balance of Power within the NHS* (DoH, 2001). The emphasis is on more extensive joint working with a wider range of partners, in some cases with more formalised structures and systems for achieving joint aims or tackling cross-cutting issues. Local strategic partnerships will align their plans for service development with the health improvement and modernisation plan (HiMP) of the local PCTs. There is no longer a requirement on local authorities to produce a community care plan, which indicates that the HiMP, along with the JIP, is the most important of the interagency planning documents for a locality, comprising statutory, voluntary and private sector alliances.

Health action zones

Health action zones are presented as an example of partnership in action, with involvement from the NHS, local authorities, community groups and the voluntary and business sectors (DoH, 2002f). They are designed to be a catalyst for encouraging existing organisations to work together to implement seven-year programmes to reduce health inequalities in their area and promote sustainable development. Research has questioned the effectiveness of such partnerships in tackling the real needs of communities and improving clinical outcomes. Crawshaw et al. (2003) explore theoretical problems in the promotion of community as a middle ground between what they call 'statist' models of society and 'market' models of the individual, with the focus on 'place' rather than 'people' poverty failing to address the structural nature of inequality. Fixed-term funding for projects militates against capacity-building and pressure to meet nationally defined targets militates against innovation. The 26 health action zones established since 1997 comprise only 1 per cent of the total health budget, so are hardly a fair challenge to conventional forms of service delivery. In common with previous experience from other regeneration programmes, it appears that the performance management regime of the Department of Health has reinforced the primacy of vertical relationships over horizontal arrangements, although, as Barnes and Sullivan (2002, p. 95) point out, the idea of joint commissioning, pooled budgets and integrated provision has since become mainstream policy through the creation of Health Act flexibilities.

Social work in primary care

Working together in health and social care is full of paradoxes. Cooperation is necessary to produce coherent care plans, but institutional barriers to cooperation remain. 'Who will pay for what' is a question not easily resolved. Medical services on the whole emphasise cure rather than care and are unlikely to prioritise chronic needs. Poxton (2003) identifies a number of different approaches to partnership working, spanning communication, coordination, collaboration and integration. There are, however, benefits in physical proximity, such as the location of social work teams in hospitals and social workers based in GP surgeries (DoH, 1994b). Early research suggested that psychiatrists and GPs had been disappointed by the community care reforms and had not seen the hoped-for expansion of choice in the provision of services (BMA, 1994). Amongst GPs, disillusionment was particularly marked in the provision of mental health services, although they identified a lack of appropriate information as a general deficit in community care. Social workers should not assume that GPs are aware of what services the local authority has available and the eligibility criteria employed. The involvement of GPs in care planning was also confused; GPs were often unsure about whether they were being asked solely to provide medical information or whether they were seen as people who could express an opinion on the viability of a care plan and were expected to have an active role in its implementation. Clarification of role therefore appears to merit further consideration. GPs were also not commonly provided with copies of the care plan; satisfaction increased the more this was done. Seeing other professionals as active partners in community care is crucial for multidisciplinary working. The development of a primary care-led NHS means that collaboration on the ground between the primary care team and social workers is even more important for the development not only of clinical pathways, but for increasing opportunities to avoid duplication and develop a whole systems approach through the use of single assessments (Audit Commission, 2002a).

Lymbery and Millward (2000) describe a history of social work attachments, to GPs' surgeries in particular, in the years preceding community care to illustrate that this is not a new development. Ratoff (1973) identified that, in those settings, social workers have the opportunity to perform valued 'diagnostic', 'liaison' and 'therapeutic' functions. Evaluating particular projects set up in Nottinghamshire, Lymbery and Millward noted a more effective use of resources, with the seconded social workers being able to deal with a greater volume of referrals, as well as better communication and an improvement in response times. The number of referrals of black service users in particular increased during the life of these projects. Working alongside GPs and primary care staff also gave social workers an enhanced professional role, leading to a more rounded assessment of need and better coordination of complex interactions. However, there were predicted tensions, notably the disparity for users between the universalism of healthcare services and the employment of strict eligibility criteria for social care. Fundamentally of concern, however, was the prospect of unconditional collaboration without a social model of health. Kharicha et al. (2004) also express concern that, while collaborative or joint working between social services and primary healthcare continues to rise up the policy agenda, current policy is not based on soundly evaluated evidence of benefit, either in terms of user and carer satisfaction or outcomes for patients, as opposed to processes experienced by professionals.

Similarly, in a study of integrated health and social care teams based in GP practices in a rural area of southwest England, Brown et al. (2003) found that there was little measurable impact of integration on clinical outcomes, or on older service users' ability to remain living in the community, although there was some improvement in the efficiency with which referrals were handled. The researchers found that 'users had little interest in who organised or delivered their services as long as they received what they felt they were entitled to' (p. 93). What was of most importance was the quality of the relationships they had with the service providers. In the teams under evaluation, separate professional line management and separate budgeting arrangements meant that team meetings were used largely for cross-referrals. Although this is a negative finding in terms of integration, it is positive in terms of the acceptability to service users of joint assessments, as predicated by the NSF for older people (see Chapter 12).

Continuing care

The division of responsibility between health and social care for continuing care needs continues to be controversial. In October 2003, nine members of the original (1999) Royal Commission on Long Term Care issued a statement asking the government to consider again the situation of older people who might be struggling inappropriately at home because they cannot afford the care they need, whilst others are bitter at the enforced loss of their home, and the dignity that goes with it, to pay for care (Royal Commission on Long Term Care, 2003). Other recommendations of the Royal Commission have been implemented:

■ the extension of direct payments to those over 65
■ the three-month disregard of the value of the home to allow for a period of rehabilitation in a residential care setting
■ the establishment of a National Care Standards Commission (now the CSCI) to monitor trends and set national benchmarks
■ the pooling of budgets for health and social care.

Registered nursing care contributions also quantify NHS responsibilities within care homes, following the exclusion of nursing care from local authority responsibilities under section 49 of the Health and Social Care Act 2001. An NSF on long-term conditions is also under construction, which will specifically address the needs of people with neurological conditions, brain or spinal injury, whose condition may be deteriorating, but who may also have needs for episodes of acute care. The fundamental question of whether the state should pay for all the long-term care needs of vulnerable adults in whatever setting is still unresolved.

Prior to April 1996, there was no compulsion on health authorities to state explicitly their policies on continuing care (Wistow, 1996). Guidance issued in 1995 (DoH, 1995b), however, required all health authorities to formulate policies for the continuing care of all adults and children in their area other than those suffering from mental illness. Crucially, this service will be free at the point of delivery. The most controversial facet of a continuing care policy is deciding who will remain in a NHS-funded bed and who will be referred on for assessment for nursing home or residential care (Henwood et al., 1997). The guidance is clear that this should be a decision taken only after consultation with all relevant parties (including the multidisciplinary team) and according to publicly available criteria. New guidance on continuing care (DoH, 2001j) sets out the parameters within which local guidance is to be developed. These are:

■ continuing care is defined as care provided by the NHS beyond the acute phase of illness or rehabilitation
■ the setting of the care should not be the sole or main determinant of eligibility
■ local eligibility criteria should be based on the nature, complexity, intensity or unpredictability of healthcare needs
■ patients who require palliative care and whose prognosis is that they are likely to die in the near future should be able to choose to remain in NHS-funded accommodation. Applications of time limits for this care are not appropriate.

The *Coughlan* judgment (McDonald, 2004) is still an authority for the premise that social care in this context is that which is 'incidental or ancillary' to the provision of accommodation. That case concerned an unsuccessful attempt to close an NHS facility and redesignate the care provided as social care. Clearly, the majority of those in need of nursing care alone will not be included in the definition of continuing care eligibility. However, the intensity of an individual's healthcare needs as well as their complexity should be taken into account. A review procedure has been made available for patients, or their carers, challenging the applicability of the continuing care criteria in individual cases. The role of social workers is not to explain or justify the application of the criteria, but they may usefully contribute to the assessment, particularly where rejection as unsuitable by one or more care homes is given as a criterion for continuing care, or where discharge to the community would be unsafe, given knowledge of the patient's previous functioning at home. Continuing care policies will equally apply to someone whose condition deteriorates in nursing home care and who should then be regarded as the responsibility of the NHS.

The health service ombudsman's special report of 2003 on NHS funding for long-term care (accessible at http://www.ombudsman.org.uk) prompted the Department of Health to ask strategic health authorities and PCTs to review decisions that they had made since 1996 to identify other patients who had wrongly been asked to pay for their care. Of the four cases considered in the report, two concerned patients with dementia, one concerned a woman severely disabled following several strokes and another concerned a delay in applying the criteria so as to enable a terminally ill woman to move closer to her family. In a later investigation (the Pointon case), the ombudsman held that the assessment for continuing care was inadequate because it failed to take into account Mr Pointon's psychological needs as a person with dementia and the needs of his wife as his carer. The application of the continuing care criteria also penalised people like Mrs Pointon who needed respite care at home, within a package of direct payments, rather than in a hospital setting.

Hospital discharge

Between 1979 and 1989, the number of available hospital beds per 1,000 population fell from 7.4 to 5.7. The average length of stay in acute specialisms fell from 9.4 to 6.4 days (DoH/SSI, 1993). By the time community care was introduced, therefore, more people were leaving hospital more quickly than 20 years previously. One in five people over the age of 65 are admitted to hospital in any one year: they occupy two-thirds of the available beds and account for half of the total growth in admissions (3.5 per cent annually). The issue of hospital discharge is therefore largely one which relates to provision for older people whose admission to acute hospital care is predominantly unplanned (DoH, 2003d; Glasby, 2003).

Discharge from hospital is a time when emotional as well as physical needs must be addressed; an assessment which focuses only on functional capacity will ignore the effect of a hospital admission on the patient's self-confidence (Horne, 1999). Hospital authorities tend to emphasise the 'safe' discharge based on assessment of medical risks. The aim instead should be to secure a 'good discharge' – one that is planned, acceptable to the patient and enduring. Neill and Williams (1992) found that two out of three of the hospital discharges of elderly patients they followed through were flawed by a lack of attention to detail, such as adequate transport arrangements or notification to friends and neighbours of the discharge plan. Deficiencies in discharge arrangements were still marked three months later at follow-up, where a high correlation was found with depression. Assessments of people's ability to cope supported only by low levels of domiciliary care was also found to be overoptimistic. Proper monitoring and review of arrangements was critical.

Quality assurance arrangements entered into by hospital trusts and social services authorities have for some time provided for minimum response times to a request from ward staff or consultant for a community care assessment. The costs of getting it wrong include:

- a poor service to patients, and unnecessarily slow recovery
- GPs not knowing what has happened to their patients
- social services staff receiving inappropriate referrals
- disputes breaking out
- unplanned readmissions
- a general waste of resources
- the risk of bad publicity on bed-blocking. (Giller and Tutt, 1995)

Many of the issues which arise in hospital discharge will also be relevant to patients presenting at A&E departments who are not subsequently admitted but who are referred on to community services including those who live out of area. Specialist hospital discharge schemes have been developed in some areas; these have been seen to offer a timely and well-integrated service but need to be planned as an overall policy, lest they increase inequity of provision and become overburdened by an inability to move people on to adequate longer term provision. Marks (1994) described hospital discharge provision as a 'patchwork quilt', despite jointly agreed discharge arrangements between health and social services departments being made a precondition from 1990 onwards for the payment of the special transitional grant transfer funding from the social security system to local authorities.

The House of Commons Health Committee (2002) found that in the second quarter of 2001, 7,000 people of all ages were awaiting discharge from hospital, costing the NHS around £720 million. This focus on performance indicators within the acute hospital care sector has led to a legislative definition of 'bed-blocking' – delayed discharges – and the introduction of penalties against social services authorities. By a complex process of notification, the 'responsible NHS body' (NHS trust or PCT in England) or local health board (in Wales) informs the relevant social services body that 'it considers that it is unlikely to be safe to discharge the patient from hospital unless one or more community care services or carers services is made available' (s.2 Community Care (Delayed Discharges) Act 2003). The social services authority will then carry out an assessment and decide which, if any, services are to be made available. The responsible NHS body then gives notice of the day on which it proposes to discharge the patient, but the notice can be as little as three days (s.5). The liability of the social services authority to make delayed discharge (or reimbursement) payments will then arise, but only if the reason for the delay is that the agreed community care or carer's service has not been made available. The whole process is predicated on medical notions of risk (the 'safe' discharge), rather than social notions of the 'good' discharge. It is likely to increase pressure to condense assessments, and will also change the working patterns of hospital social workers in order to cover 'out of hours' discharges and may damage good working relationships (Glasby, 2003). A new edition of the *Hospital Discharge Workbook* was published by the DoH in 2003 entitled *Discharge from Hospital: Pathway, Process and Practice*. The guidance emphasises that effective hospital discharge depends on a whole systems approach, including housing authorities, the active involvement of patients and carers and the identification of vulnerable individuals on admission. The guidance also recommends the appointment of 'care coordinators' at ward level and integrated discharge planning teams. It is important, however, that all patients should be assessed for a period of rehabilitation before any permanent decisions on care options are made (Nocon and Baldwin, 1998). A study by SCIE (2004) into the impact of the 2003 Act found that delayed discharges had almost halved between October 2003 and January 2004 but that there was a wide variation across the country in terms of reliance on residential care and readmission rates.

Intermediate care

Intermediate care is described by the Department of Health (2001k) as an innovatory stage between acute care and long-term care, designed to either prevent admission to hospital or facilitate discharge. It is intended to be short term, that is, for a period of two to six weeks and may be provided either by the NHS or social services authorities, but is free at the point of use up to the six-week period. A number of service models are possible, including:

- Rapid response
- Hospital at home
- Residential rehabilitation
- Supported discharge
- Day rehabilitation.

The idea of intermediate care was included in the 1997 NHS plan and the target of 2,400 more beds by 2003–4 has been met. Since the evidence base is limited, intermediate care is something of a leap of faith and at the present time its status is unclear; is it a way of freeing beds or is it a support for the independence of older people (Petch, 2003)?

The variety and complexity of intermediate care services has been surveyed by Martin et al. (2004). The configuration of intermediate care services appears to respond to gaps in existing service provision and can range from low-level social rehabilitation to intensive therapeutic intervention following an acute medical admission. The King's Fund has an extensive literature on rehabilitation and intermediate care (accessible at http://www.kingsfund.org.uk). The introduction of a new range of services, bridging hospital and home, has implications for established hospital discharge practices, including predischarge home visits that are commonly undertaken in advance of a return home from acute care, particularly for frail older people. But, as Mountain and Pighills (2003) point out, an anxious assurance that discharge is safe in the short term does not guarantee the ability to cope in the longer term.

The social worker in a healthcare setting

The role of the social worker in a hospital setting post-community care was examined by Davies and Connolly (1995). They found that personal factors such as approachability, good timekeeping and responsiveness were valued more highly by medical and clinical staff than social work skills. However, those who valued the social worker as a professional, with a distinct body of knowledge and skills different from their own, were more realistically satisfied with outcomes than were those who saw the social worker as a technician – able, or unable, to respond to a request for a particular service. Hospital social workers may feel marginalised compared to fieldwork colleagues and have a less strong management structure. Their role in bringing services to people who might not otherwise come to the attention of social care agencies is, however, seen as critical by McLeod (1996). Department of Health (DoH, 2003d) research on the discharge of hospital patients also found that both patients and carers were overwhelmingly grateful for the support provided by hospital social workers. How to maintain autonomy despite continued healthcare requirements is discussed by McWilliams et al. (1994); central to this is a patient-centred approach based on the individual's goals, aspirations and sense of purpose within a larger life context. Hence the importance within the social work task of a holistic but person-centred assessment. Research in the US also found that early and frequent social worker interventions were associated with significantly shorter hospital stays, for non-medical reasons (Fillit et al., 1992).

Five practice elements may be identified as central to hospital social work: interdisciplinary collaboration; assessment; communication between the hospital and the community; networking and negotiation; and using financial acumen. The discharge planning process had already attained pre-eminence; but Davies and Connolly (1995a) found that there were two areas of dissonance: counselling and clients' rights. Counselling in hospital was seen not primarily as a social work task, but one which was also undertaken by nursing staff. Indeed, the processing framework of the NHSCCA 1990 (as it was perceived to be) undervalued the need for counselling. In terms of client rights, there was conflict between medical notions of safety and seeing that the wishes of the patient were followed, although social workers attached to specialist units tended to have their role of representing patients' interests more commonly recognised as legitimate. Ahulu (1995), however, counsels against centring concern over issues of dependency and control only in the community; he sees these as equally relevant to hospital care. It is therefore false to assume that vulnerable people living in hospitals or institutions present no problems and that difficulties only arise when such people are discharged into the community. Vulnerable people in hospital and institutions deserve the same level of concern and attention advocated for those living at home.

McLeod et al. (2003) have researched the contribution that social workers located in hospital A&E departments can make to the care of older people. Thirty per cent of A&E departments now have a social worker as part of the team. The older people interviewed in McLeod et al.'s research rated most highly the following types of assistance: help with negotiating the demands of attending

A&E itself; help with accessing social services; and easier access to placements in intermediate healthcare. Nevertheless, access to a social worker was limited by inadequate resourcing and reflected the general position of a disproportionately low rate of referrals from minority ethnic groups. Also, the effectiveness of the social worker's input at A&E was undermined by the shortage of longer term resources. Delays in starting services, inadequate services to meet need and a shortage of interim care placements were identified as risk factors for readmission to hospital. There was also considerable evidence of continuing and significant unmet healthcare needs. To an extent, therefore, the intransigent nature of these older patients' healthcare needs undermine the basic premise of the placement: that social care could adequately compensate for real healthcare needs, instead of being inextricably interlinked with them.

Mental health

Services for people who are mentally ill exemplify the two sides of community care: preventive work with people in the community to maintain them in the community, and the legacy of the movement to discharge people from the large psychiatric hospitals into the community. Health authorities remain the lead authorities in the provision of services for the mentally ill. This in itself has led to anomalies within the system of community care. Concerned by reports of inadequate care being provided for patients discharged from long-stay hospitals, the government issued guidance to all health authorities on the care programme approach (CPA) (DoH, 1990a), on the care of people referred to specialist psychiatric services. This system thus predated the system of care management introduced in the wake of the NHSCCA 1990. The two systems continued to run in parallel; one health authority-led, the other local authority-led, but both would often concentrate on the same people. The CPA focuses on the appointment of a care coordinator (who may come from any discipline) to oversee the care of the patient in hospital and the community. A fuller explanation of the CPA and its relationship to care management was provided by the Department of Health in *Building Bridges* (DoH, 1995); it stressed that the two systems are based on the same principles and are capable of being integrated through a consistently applied initial screening process to ensure the most effective deployment of professional skills on a cross-agency basis. Partnership with the voluntary and private sector was also to be encouraged (DoH, 1997).

Public concern over inadequate follow-up of previously detained patients and uncoordinated involvement by different professionals found its expression in the report into the death of Christopher Clunis (DoH, 1994). As a consequence, supervision registers were introduced to monitor those patients seen as a risk to themselves or others in the community. There were considerable discrepancies in the operation of such registers and the social work role was unclear (Bird and Davies, 1996). A later development has been the introduction of a power of supervised discharge (but not treatment) in the community by the Supervision of Patients in the Community Act 1995. There the role of the social worker is clearly subordinated to that of the responsible medical officer (RMO), as it is the RMO and not the social worker who makes the application for a supervised discharge order; a reversal of the roles undertaken when the patient is sectioned under the Mental Health Act 1983. Both supervision registers and supervised discharge emphasise the control rather than the care aspect of community services. In the event, however, these powers have been little used because of a general refocusing of the CPA itself, and the category of supervised discharge is likely to be abolished in the near future.

The CPA was modernised in 1999 to focus on individuals with severe and enduring mental illness (DoH, 1999a). All health and social services authorities were required to appoint a 'lead officer' to ensure the development of an integrated approach across all agencies and services. The CPA was widened to include 'all those people who are under the care of the secondary mental health services regardless of setting', not just those about to be discharged from hospital, and was streamlined into:

- *Standard CPA:* for individuals who require the support or intervention of only one agency or discipline, or pose no danger to themselves or others, and who will not be at high risk if they lose contact with services.
- *Enhanced CPA:* for individuals who have multiple needs, including those who also have a drugs/alcohol problem. This category includes those at risk and those hard to engage and requires crisis and contingency plans.

The Mental Health Act 1983 continues to provide the legislative framework for the compulsory admission to hospital of those suffering from mental disorder, although section 131 of the Act maintains that informal admission should be the norm. The code of practice under the Act sets out principles for the application of the Act, placing an emphasis on the patient as an individual with rights and the need for different agencies to cooperate. The CPA provides the structure within which services are delivered and the application of the Act is limited to the least detrimental alternative that is compatible with ensuring the patient's own health or safety or the safety of other people. In 1999, proposals were made for the reform of the Mental Health Act (DoH, 1999b), but they have been controversial and legislation based on them has been delayed. Matters of contention have been:

- the wider definition of mental disorder
- the introduction of compulsory treatment within the community
- reference to a mental health tribunal to confirm care plans rather than as a review mechanism
- the detention of people with severe personality disorders
- the proposed extension of the sectioning power beyond approved social workers to other approved mental health professionals.

Proposals to reform the law dealing with mental incapacity have been separated out from the original consultation, and are dealt with in Chapter 8. The impact of community care policies more generally on people with mental health problems and an analysis of the NSF for mental health can be found in Chapter 12. Mental health services continue to epitomise the care/control debate in health and social care and the conflicts between medical models of treatment and social support for marginalised individuals.

Future developments

The use of Health Act flexibilities has enabled the mainstreaming of collaboration arrangements to take place, but the most recent practice development in preventive work is designed to evaluate the use not of social work, but nursing skills. The Evercare Programme developed in the USA has been a significant development in improving quality of life for vulnerable older people with chronic conditions (Evercare, 2004). This is achieved by targeting intensive care management by healthcare professionals at older people most at risk. There have been nine pilots in the UK within PCTs. The implementation phase began in April 2003 through to August 2004. In the USA, hospital admissions for over-65s on the programme were reduced by 50 per cent. In the UK, the target population was the 3 per cent of the over-65s who were responsible for 35 per cent of the unplanned admissions for that age group. The project was designed to identify this previously 'invisible' population, only 24 per cent of whom were active on the district nurse caseloads and 35 per cent of whom were on social services caseloads. In many ways, Evercare replicates the original community care demonstration projects in the UK, but transfers the practice to a primary care health-led setting.

Recent developments in the NHS seem likely to roll out the Evercare principles within primary care. Chapter 3 of *The NHS Improvement Plan* (DoH, 2004a) begins to shift the focus from acute care to people with long-term chronic conditions. Although only 5 per cent of the population, people with chronic conditions account for 40 per cent of NHS spending. These are conditions such as diabetes, asthma, arthritis, skin diseases and depression that can be controlled but not necessarily cured. The focus is on 'personalised care' for three identified groups of patients:

- Those who can manage their own conditions as 'expert patients'
- Those who need more proactive support
- A smaller group with particularly complex needs who require a 'case management' approach with more active and specialist care.

Expert patient pilots in PCTs across the country will be rolled out nationally in 2008, supported by incentives for preventive work in the new GP contract and guidance from NICE. 'Disease management' will facilitate better monitoring of patients in the second category. Case management builds on the Evercare model for all patients with three or more long-term health problems (15 per cent of the total). It is anticipated that every PCT will offer this model of care by 2008.

A number of principles are set out for links with social care. These are:

- Social care needs are person-centred and personalised and also require people to be involved in the design and delivery of services
- Proactive services should stop problems happening and help people to maintain independence and existing networks of support
- Social care commissioning and provision should be further integrated with healthcare
- Social care is critical to prevention; it includes effective home care, better transport, housing, leisure and community networks.

Changes are also anticipated in the wake of the White Paper on public health (DoH, 2004c), which addresses environmental issues as well as individual prevention strategies to develop a holistic, community-based approach to identifying and meeting healthcare needs, albeit with a continuing emphasis on personal responsibility and health promotion.

Concluding comments

This chapter looked at the changing roles of stakeholders in the provision of community care and movements in the balance of power and influence in its operation. There has been a steady increase in the role of the NHS as the primary mover in this area, but little hard evidence that working alongside social care has led to real collaboration or a shared philosophy of care. There are still important border issues to be addressed concerning continuing care and delayed discharges, in particular. The concept of intermediate care is also in need of further study to establish itself with a proper rehabilitative focus rather than as a service to ease pressure on the acute or community sectors. There have also been important changes within the NHS to shift the balance in favour of primary care because of its role in commissioning services and strategic importance in developing community-based responses to healthcare needs. The mixed economy of care that was a signature feature of social care in the early 1990s looks set to become an important aspect of healthcare in the next decade, as the public sector diversifies and increasingly contracts with the private healthcare sector. This issue is further discussed in Chapter 12. Chapter 11 looks at another aspect of interagency working – the interface between social care and housing.

PAUSE AND REFLECT

Find a copy of the continuing care policy which operates in your area. In what circumstances would the policy apply to:

1. George Adams, aged 58, a patient in a specialist stroke unit within a general hospital, who has had a severe stroke and needs PEG feeding and hoisting.
2. Edith Bowers, aged 85, a resident in a nursing home, who has multi-infarct dementia and is aggressive towards both staff and fellow residents.

CASE STUDY

Aftercare

Philip Lee is 26 years old and his ethnicity is Chinese. He has a diagnosis of paranoid schizophrenia and has had a number of hospital admissions in the past. Most recently, he has been admitted under section 3 of the Mental Health Act 1983 for treatment, after threatening to throw himself off a bridge. Philip lives with his mother, who is willing to have him at home, but feels she needs help in looking after him. Philip's condition deteriorates when he fails to take his medication.

What legal provisions would apply in anticipation of Philip's discharge from hospital? What sort of support might assist him and his family?

FURTHER READING

Allen, I. (2001) *Social Care and Health: A New Deal?* London: Policy Studies Institute.
Charts recent changes in the organisation of the NHS and examines the concept of partnership working between health and social care.

Bradley, G. and Manthorpe, J. (eds) (2000) *Working on the Fault Line*. Birmingham: Venture Press.
Describes the social role in a range of healthcare settings, explaining opportunities and conflicts in interagency collaboration.

Glasby, J. and Littlechild, R. (2004) *The Health and Social Care Divide: The Experiences of Older People* (rev 2nd edn). Bristol: Policy Press.
Traces the history of collaboration between the NHS and social care, with chapters on hospital discharge, rehabilitation and intermediate care, continuing care and mental health services. Includes extended case studies, policy digests and discussion of practice issues. Clearly written and extensively referenced.

CHAPTER 11

Social and Housing Needs

Introduction

Integrated service provision also requires that housing issues are taken into account alongside social care and healthcare. This chapter looks at interagency collaboration and how assessments are carried out for a range of people with housing needs. These range from owner-occupiers whose property is in need of adaptation due to disability, to the housing needs of ex-prisoners and provision for homeless families. *Supporting People* (ODPM, 2003) has separated out the bricks and mortar element of housing benefit from the funding and provision of support needs through interagency partnerships. This may mean that people with lower level needs who would not otherwise meet eligibility criteria for community care services may now be supported. At the other end of the spectrum of need, this chapter also looks at good practice in the transition to residential care and the location of residential provision within a definition of housing need. Housing and its association with community care services is increasingly being recognised as vital to maintaining people within the community. It is not only public sector housing that has an essential contribution to make; given that the majority of people in the UK are now owner-occupiers, properly utilising and maintaining private sector housing is important as well. Homelessness, whether hidden or overt, may be a trigger for the provision of community care services or a consequence of their absence. There is a further link between deficiencies in housing services and admissions to long-term care. In the continuum of need, therefore, housing has a vital role to play.

Types of housing

Means and Smith (1994, p. 166) begin from the premise that:

> Community care policy in the UK is based on the belief that nearly everyone prefers to live in ordinary housing rather than in institutions, because institutions lack the capacity to be a home.

'Home' in this sense means more than bricks and mortar, insofar as it defines the sense of self, particularly if there is continuity over time, by meeting fundamental attachment needs. This is why relocation for older people especially can be so traumatic, in circumstances when there is little choice over whether, and to where, the move should be made (Willcocks et al., 1987). People's housing needs, in this sense, will be particular to them as individuals and need to be recognised as such in any joint assessment. Freedom of choice, however, is often limited by policy decisions, as, for example, in the operation of housing benefit rules (Griffiths, 1997) or by administrative processes, such as the allocation of funding for adaptations to property.

Housing policy since 1979 has supported:

- an increase in owner-occupation
- the diminution of the local authority's own housing stock
- the expansion of housing association provision
- the development of supported housing
- differentials in the receipt of public assistance through the housing benefit scheme.

These policy trends were well established in their own right, before the introduction of the system of community care. Integration of the two systems, however, received little attention. Arguably, this lack of integration has been a major defect of community care policy.

Owner-occupation

Levels of home ownership in the first decade of this century include substantial numbers of older people (Means, 1997). Redundancy and early retirement will mean that one-third of owner-occupiers aged 65–74 in 2011 will still have a mortgage to pay (Hancock, 1998). Middle-class impoverishment related to housing is likely to become an important issue for social policy in the future. The implication of the trend towards owner-occupation is that substantial amounts of capital are tied up in bricks and mortar. A tension is then created between the potential of that capital, as inheritance to be passed down the generations, and its availability, as a resource for meeting the care needs of the present generation – particularly when admission to residential care is being contemplated. How this dilemma is related to current charging policies is discussed in Chapter 9. Social workers may have to deal with very real feelings of disappointment and loss when assets have to be cashed in order to meet long-term care needs.

Owner-occupation brings with it a responsibility for maintenance and repair. Disrepair is a major issue for low-income owner-occupiers (Mackintosh et al., 1990). The majority of those living in housing which is lacking in basic amenities or in need of considerable repair are older people. The disabled facilities grant, which was introduced in 1990 and designed to enable properties to be made more suitable for the needs of disabled residents, has not been supported significantly through funding, whilst early hospital discharge and the introduction of EU regulations regarding lifting have increased demand (Heywood and Smart, 1996). Social services and housing departments have a joint responsibility for housing adaptations, such as the installation of lifts and showers, under the Chronically Sick and Disabled Persons Act 1970 (Mandelstam, 1997). The current legislation on grants is the Housing Grants, Construction and Regeneration Act 1996. Under this Act, the housing authority must approve grant applications which will facilitate access, make the dwelling safe or improve the heating system for the benefit of a disabled person. The housing authority is required to consult with the social services authority, usually through an occupational therapy assessment, in deciding whether the relevant works are necessary and appropriate and then decides whether it is reasonable and practicable to carry them out within a financial limit for grants of £25,000. Disabled facilities grants are the only mandatory grants to remain under the 1996 Act, although local authorities have a discretion to provide other types of financial support to improve property. Means-testing takes into account not only the income of the applicant but also that of other persons occupying the house.

Local authority housing

A seminal feature of housing policy in the decade prior to the enactment of community care was the introduction by Part V of the Housing Act 1985 of the 'right to buy' legislation. Although such a right also extends to tenants of housing associations and housing action trusts, it is the local authority housing stock which has been irretrievably depleted by the right to buy. There are, however, certain exemptions to the right to buy legislation for specialist housing, which preserves this as a resource for the public sector. On an individual level, one consequence of exercising the right to buy is that housing benefit is no longer available. At a collective level, it means that public subsidy is no longer available through bricks and mortar, but by means-tested financial assessment for those who remain council tenants.

Housing associations

Alongside policy developments in council house sales have come cutbacks in the housing investment programmes of local authorities (Malpas and Means, 1993). The gap was expected to be filled by housing associations as the main providers of new rented housing. Housing associations are quasi-autonomous organisations operating under the general control of the Housing Corporation. The 1988 Housing Act introduced a new funding regime for housing associations which provided only part of their capital finance from public funds, but required them to raise the majority of their funding on the open market. One effect of this has been to push up rents (Means and Smith, 1994). Another effect has been to remove much responsibility for housing development out of direct democratic control and create an internal market within the public and not-for-profit sectors. Generally, a proportion of housing association lets are reserved for local authority nominees from the housing list.

Specialist housing and supported housing

The growth of specialist and supported housing schemes, and their seeming appropriateness within a system of community care, should not obscure the vital role still to be played by mainstream housing. To do so is to the detriment of both housing and social care agencies; the former because tenants who are in need of supportive services may have those needs overlooked because they are 'mainstream' and not 'special', and the latter because they may ignore the normalisation potential of mainstream housing and a package of services, as opposed to specialist provision. Special needs housing has nevertheless been a major growth area, which even in the 1980s accounted for one-third of all housing completions (Stewart and Stewart, 1993).

The earliest and most common type of specialist housing to emerge was sheltered housing for older people, which now covers a wide range of tenure arrangements (to buy, rent or own), and varying degrees of support therein. Support may range from on- or off-site warden provision to 'very sheltered housing' schemes where personal and domestic care as well as housing is provided. There is evidence that residents of existing sheltered housing schemes are becoming more frail and are tending to remain there (Watson and Cooper, 1992). On the other hand, Tinker (1989) found that some specialist housing schemes were hard to let, and one-quarter of the sample in that research would have preferred to remain in their original home with more domiciliary support.

A report by Values into Action was critical of schemes which combined as a package housing and social care (Collins, 1996). In the case of people with learning disabilities, such schemes were seen as less likely to respect their rights as citizens to make individual choices than where the two functions were clearly separated. Written agreements between user and provider were used not to guarantee rights as tenants, but explicitly to support the unit's operating policy and focus concerns on the user. The legal position of some housing with care schemes is unclear. Whether or not such schemes are required to register as care homes may depend not just on whether tenants have their own front door, but whether they have been able to exercise a free choice in moving to this type of accommodation, even if a separate company provides the care (Clements, 2004).

Oldman (2000) looked at the qualitative differences and similarities between housing with care and care home accommodation. She found that newer forms of sheltered housing, incorporating the provision of meals and domiciliary services, were accommodating people with similar levels of frailty to those living in care homes. However, in terms of structure, the boundaries between the two types of provision are rigid. Because of the different funding structure, residents of sheltered housing schemes have a far higher disposable income. It is also easier to provide services according to independent living philosophies to people who 'have their own front door'. The enhanced sheltered housing schemes also received a hidden subsidy from relatives' informal caring, whereas in residential care, relatives usually took on the role of visitor only. The principal benefits of moving into very sheltered accommodation were an improved quality of life and an enhanced feeling of both physical and psychological security. Schemes which based admissions policy on dependency levels only were seen to be in danger of hampering the concept of a lively community (preferred by residents), but were also the schemes most successful in limiting transfer to residential care, hence supporting the argument that they could reduce reliance on or even replace care home provision.

Interagency collaboration

Interagency collaboration is once again seen as the key to successful community care, both at a strategic and individual level. This includes addressing health as well as social care needs within a housing context (Arblaster et al., 1996). There has been little evidence that formal care management is offering a more coordinated response. Real barriers can be created by social services departments' eligibility criteria being pitched at such a high level, with serious shortfalls in care support for people with medium and low levels of need. The housing allocation process itself, with limited choice and short response times, assumes that people are poised to move and can make a rapid response to a given offer. Yet there are not necessarily systems in place to help people to deal with the practical and emotional difficulties of moving house. Lack of skills in money management and running a household were identified by Hudson et al. (1996) as a major barrier to people moving into new accommodation. Users are often fitted into a limited range of options, rather than being given significant choice. This raises particular issues of anti-discriminatory practice when what is on offer is plainly unsuitable.

Research into the housing and mental healthcare needs of Asian people found that housing for Asian people with mental health problems was in many cases inappropriate and often added to their difficulties in daily living (Radia, 1996). Myths and stereotypes of Asian people, particularly the ability and willingness of families to provide care, continued to dominate the thinking of both policy-makers and professionals. There was a shortage of specialist residential projects and an absence of good financial advice. Support services were inadequate and sometimes of poor quality. Age Concern, Scotland also found that few community care plans considered the special needs of older people with mental health problems, or how they might be provided with more suitable housing (Adams and Wilson, 1996). This is despite statistical evidence that 25 per cent of over-55s on local authority waiting lists cited mental disorder as a reason for seeking priority in rehousing. For this group, good housing brought physical as well as psychological benefits; conversely, the impact of poor housing on a psychologically frail person could be disproportionate. Given the importance of social support and the overriding need to avoid loneliness and hostility from neighbours, shared living – with careful attention paid to the mix of residents – was found to have real advantages.

The relationship between poor health, disability and housing allocation is complex. Advice from the Scottish Federation of Housing Associations, for example, is that weightings given to medical factors must be 'appropriate', but need not be overriding. Despite the amount of hope and energy expended in obtaining evidence for medical priority, other factors, such as the absence of security of tenure and lack of basic amenities, are likely to be of overriding importance. The trend in medical priority allocations is towards self-assessment, with endorsement by GPs at the appeal stage (SCFA, 1995). Certainly, visible physical or mobility problems attract priority far more readily than psychological/mental health considerations. Indeed, many housing associations have chosen not to give points for anxiety or depression not requiring current treatment, given the generalised nature of these conditions. Asthma is another condition which, contrary to popular belief, is not a high priority unless there is overwhelming evidence that particular characteristics of the property severely exacerbate the condition. HIV/AIDS are often treated as 'special lets' outside the main points system, given the need for confidentiality and the deteriorating nature of the conditions. For their part, social workers find housing problems among the most difficult to handle, 'possibly because the solutions are so obvious yet so hard to achieve' (Stewart and Stewart, 1993). The consequences of not dealing effectively with a housing problem may mean greater deterioration in the health, financial and relationship difficulties of those concerned. Section 47 of the NHSCCA 1990 requires SSDs to consider housing needs, thus highlighting the issue as one component of a comprehensive assessment of need; housing need in itself cannot be divorced from whatever else is going on in people's lives.

Supporting People

A desire to end the complexity of different systems for supporting vulnerable residents and a desire to separate housing funding from care services led to the creation of the *Supporting People* programme (ODPM, 2003) as one of the major recent innovations in housing policy. The *Supporting People* programme was originally launched in March 1999 by the then Department of Transport, Local Government and the Regions and is now within the remit of the Office of the Deputy Prime Minister (ODPM). It aims to separate out the bricks and mortar element of housing benefit (see Chapter 9) from the provision of support services. Councils, involving housing and social services, administer the new funding framework in partnership with the NHS, the Probation Service, service user groups and support agencies. Interagency cooperation is therefore placed at a premium and differentials in sources of support are reduced. The programme 'offers vulnerable people the opportunity to improve their quality of life by providing a stable environment which enables greater independence' (ODPM, 2003). *Supporting People* teams have been created on a local basis to coordinate the provision of support services to a range of vulnerable people following assessment.

Supporting People is rightly seen as part of the continuum of provision and charging for services which extends from accommodation costs, through support and personal care to nursing care (Griffiths, 2000). *Supporting People* introduces a 'third way', which may offer a real alternative to residential care for people with considerable support needs, but which also enables short-term preventive work to be done with homeless young people, people with mental health problems, those recovering from drug and alcohol misuse and ex-offenders. *Supporting People* therefore enables vulnerable people who might not meet the eligibility criteria for a social work service to be supported in the community in a non-stigmatising way. The support provided can enable people to retain their accommodation in circumstances which might otherwise lead to homelessness or institutionalisation.

Homelessness

The legislative framework within which housing departments work determines that their culture is a 'gatekeeping' one rather than one based on need (Cowan,

1995). Part VII of the Housing Act 1996, which deals with homelessness, is a good example of this. In order to qualify fully for assistance under the Act, an individual applicant must satisfy the following criteria:

- that he is homeless
- that he is in priority need
- that he is not homeless intentionally
- that he has a local connection with the housing authority to which he applies.

The definition of 'homelessness' is wider that that of 'rooflessness'; persons living in crisis accommodation, refuges or night shelters are homeless, as are people who have accommodation that it would be unreasonable for them to occupy, for example because they are threatened with domestic or other forms of violence. A person who is threatened with homelessness will qualify if he or she is likely to become homeless within 28 days. An example of totally unsuitable accommodation would be that which is overcrowded or unsuitable for a physically disabled occupant. An adult living with family in circumstances where he or she is not the householder may also seek to present himself or herself as homeless, if, perhaps as a result of a dispute, he or she is asked to leave. Much actual homelessness may in fact be hidden by multiple occupations or families moving in with friends. Homelessness may also be an outcome of intervention by other systems, such as unplanned admission to hospital or imprisonment.

Local authorities are obliged to provide advice and assistance to all persons who are homeless. However, it is only people who are in 'priority need' who are owed a duty by the local authority to ensure that accommodation becomes available for their occupation. Those in priority need are defined within the Housing Act 1996 as:

- pregnant women (at any stage of their pregnancy)
- persons with dependent children
- those who are homeless as a result of an emergency such as fire, flood or other disaster
- persons who are vulnerable as a result of old age, mental illness or handicap, physical disability or other special reason. In considering vulnerability due to mental or physical illness or disability, authorities should have regard to medical advice and, where appropriate, seek social services advice.

Entitlement to accommodation may, however, be lost because of a further finding that the applicant is homeless intentionally, for example by doing something which leads to his or her lawful eviction, such as causing a nuisance or not paying the rent. The behaviour concerned must, however, be deliberate; 'real financial difficulties' leading to default or circumstances where the authority has reason to believe that the applicant is incapable of managing his/her affairs, for example on account of old age, mental illness or disability, should not count as deliberate behaviour. Those who are homeless intentionally still have a right to temporary accommodation for such time as the local authority consider will give the person a reasonable opportunity of securing accommodation (normally

28 days). It is for the authority to establish intentionality, not for the applicant to disprove it.

The final hurdle to be overcome is that of 'local connection', not to be confused with that of ordinary residence under the National Assistance Act 1948. Under the homelessness legislation, a local authority may refer on a person who has no local connection with their own area, but does have a local connection with the area of another authority. Local connection can be established by prior residence, employment, family association or other special circumstances. A person who is at risk of violence in that other authority should not be referred on. If a person who is unintentionally homeless and in priority need has no local connection with the area of any housing authority in Great Britain, the duty to secure accommodation for that person rests with the authority to which application is made.

The Housing Act 1996 has been amended in a number of important respects by the Homelessness Act 2002. The 2002 Act imposes a duty on local authorities to produce a homelessness strategy involving consultation with social services authorities, but removes the obligation to maintain a housing register. Although there is no duty to provide permanent accommodation at the outset, the free-market principle contained in the 1996 Act – that the local authority owed no duty to homeless people in circumstances where there was a ready supply of private accommodation – is now abolished. Also, under the 1996 Act, the local authority's duty was limited to a two-year period – this limitation is now removed. Homeless 16–17-year-olds who are not the responsibility of social services authorities under the Children (Leaving Care) Act 2000 or section 20 of the CA 1989 are also now deemed to be in priority need. People under the age of 21 who have been in the care system may also be considered vulnerable, as may people discharged from the armed forces and ex-prisoners. Where families with children are turned away by housing departments as intentionally homeless, they are to be referred on with their consent to social services for support under the CA 1989. There has thus been an amelioration of the harshness of some aspects of the legal position in the 1990s and a greater emphasis on interagency cooperation. However, for social services authorities, this may mean that they have a higher residual duty towards vulnerable individuals and families than previously. The impact of the Human Rights Act 1998, particularly the right to respect for privacy and family life contained in Article 8 of the European Convention on Human Rights, has been felt by agencies who may have duties under either or both the CA 1989 and the NHSCCA 1990. So, for example, parents with mental health problems affected by homelessness or poor housing, or children with disabilities needing adapted properties may look to support from social services authorities as well as housing authorities for accommodation to maintain their right to family life (McDonald, 2004).

Antisocial behaviour

At the same time that amendments were being made to the homelessness legislation to support 'deserving' applicants, antisocial behaviour was being stringently sanctioned in legislation throughout the late 1990s, culminating in the

Anti-Social Behaviour Act 2003. As well as incurring penalties under criminal law, people who behave in an antisocial way towards their neighbours may find that their tenancies are demoted from secure tenancies to periodic weekly tenancies. Housing authorities including housing associations can apply for antisocial behaviour orders against tenants. Parents can be made subject to parenting orders to enforce their responsibilities for their children's behaviour. In the context of community care, there is a complex interplay between the law on antisocial behaviour and disability discrimination. People with mental health problems, for example, who are perceived as harassing their neighbours may successfully argue that they would not have behaved in such a way but for their disability. Therefore to apply sanctions against them for that behaviour is less favourable treatment than would be given to others (McDonald, 2004).

Dealing with antisocial behaviour is seen as a multiagency responsibility. There is an emphasis on community responsibility and the diversion of young people in particular from antisocial behaviour. Examples of effective practice are available on the Together website, maintained by the Home Office, at http://www.together.gov.uk. The social worker's role in dealing with antisocial behaviour is not without conflict, however. Professional dilemmas may well arise in some of the following circumstances:

- being asked to use community activities to monitor and track individuals' behaviour
- sharing this sort of information with enforcement agencies
- supporting individuals and families in conflict with other agencies, for example those threatened with eviction by housing agencies because of antisocial behaviour
- being defined in an enforcement role themselves because of the wide definition of antisocial behaviour in civil as well as criminal terms.

Ex-prisoners

The housing needs of ex-prisoners need to be addressed within both the criminal justice system and housing policy (Carlisle, 1996). Prisoners who do not find satisfactory accommodation on release are more likely to reoffend within the first 12 months than those with accommodation deemed to be 'good'. The problem is numerically large: approximately 90,000 prisoners are released into the community each year. Less than half the prisoners in Carlisle's study were able to return to their previous home. Three factors were instrumental in determining whether ex-prisoners succeeded in retaining their homes:

- quality of family relationships
- availability of housing benefit
- financial status.

The largest group to lose their housing in the community were owner-occupiers who had no financial support otherwise available to them, following a reduction in the period during which housing benefit would be paid from 52 weeks to a maximum of 13 weeks. The group most likely to be disadvantaged were single mothers. Organisational factors were also found to militate against a well-planned transition back into the community. Although probation officers within prisons were actively involved in discussing housing matters, nowhere were there written procedures or guidance relating to housing. Local authorities and housing associations would not accept onto their lists people who were in prison, although very few ex-prisoners were happy to accept hostel accommodation, even when available. There have, however, been some positive recent developments. NACRO has produced guidance for prisoners and those working with them on housing issues, which include some standard letters relating to applications and finance, and is the major voluntary organisation contracting to assess the accommodation needs of prisoners (see www.nacro.org.uk). Reporting requirements for prisoners on licence or prisoners who are being electronically monitored increase the need for suitable supportive accommodation, thus giving the issue a higher priority in terms of forward planning.

Residential care

An increasing range of accommodation now exists for people with care needs, such that the boundaries between 'home' and 'institutional' care are by no means clear-cut (Higgins, 1989). The traditional dualism between residential care and care in the community has been questioned by Jack (1998), who sees good quality residential care as necessarily having links into, and being supported by, the community within which it is located. Very sheltered housing, core and cluster schemes and shared living schemes have all developed to meet a spectrum of need. Yet the basic question remains: why should people have to change their permanent residence simply in order to obtain the services which they need (Wagner, 1988)? In other words, why cannot services be brought to the people, rather than people to the service? Housing schemes which allow people to move within the same site from very sheltered housing to residential care and then on to nursing care are one solution. Better coordination between health and social care to put together a package of care at home is another.

Concern about the overprovision and high cost of residential care was a prime incentive behind the community care changes in the early 1990s. Subsequent policy, however, has been riddled with inconsistencies to do with funding and registration requirements. There is no continuing obligation on local authorities directly to provide residential care services, and some authorities have either sold off their remaining homes or have transferred managerial responsibility to not-for-profit organisations operating as trusts. The financial implications for residents of moving into different types of residential care are discussed in Chapter 9, but residents will also be concerned about the quality of the care that they receive and how this can be assured.

Choice in residential care, whether that is choice of whether or not to enter the residential sector in the first place or choice of location, is probably still more apparent than real. Changes in the funding arrangements for residential care, with top-up funding being removed from the DSS budget to individual local authorities, were designed to ensure that no one entered residential care supported by public funding without the appropriateness of that move being assessed. Statistics themselves disguise the fact that, for most people in residential care, the decision to enter that type of care was neither a matter of free choice nor were they necessarily consulted about the decision. Relatives, friends and GPs are prime movers in the process. The challenge for the social worker (and the local authority) is how best to build on the strengths and work to overcome the negative factors which may precipitate people into residential care. Some of the factors are organisational, some are due to poor practice and some are psychosocial in origin. A number of themes emerge (Warburton, 1989):

- fears about living alone, precipitated by crisis or bereavement
- increasing impairment and disability
- a shortage of community services
- carers' stress and lack of support for carers
- poor or ineffective assessment and care management
- inadequate preparation for leaving hospital
- lack of service innovation and inflexibility
- professional and organisational concerns and interests, examples being overconcern about risk, insufficient time to allocate to assessment and the precipitate closure of continuing care beds.

Careful handling of the admission to residential care is vital; the process of giving up one's own home, leaving neighbourhood and friends and adapting to communal living may correctly be perceived as a crisis (Sinclair et al., 1990). Being given real options and a real choice, at this stage, is a good indicator of a successful outcome (Willcocks et al., 1987). Choice may be limited by availability, cost or the contracting arrangements of local authorities. If choice appears to be limited unreasonably, reference should be made to the National Assistance Act 1948 (Choice of Accommodation) Directions 1992. If a person (or their carer if that person is unable to express a preference) expresses a preference for particular accommodation (known as 'preferred accommodation') within the UK, the authority must arrange for care in that accommodation, provided that:

- the accommodation is suitable in relation to the individual's assessed need
- to do so would not cost the authority more than it would usually pay for accommodation of that type, unless the individual or a third party is willing to meet the difference in cost
- the accommodation is available
- the person in charge of the accommodation is willing to provide it, subject to the authority's usual terms and conditions for such accommodation.

The local authority that imposes a rigid ceiling on the cost of the residential care that it is willing to fund will not be interpreting this direction properly. An individual assessment of need should lead to an individual service response. Psychological needs are as important as physical needs in the assessment and the original guidance which accompanied the directions specifically referred to the need to be near family (albeit in a different part of the country) as an important need to respect; the fact that care charges may be higher in that other region is an irrelevant consideration in this respect. The scope of the directions was tested in the case of Mark Hazell, a young man with Down syndrome living in Avon, who challenged, through the complaints procedure and later by judicial review, his authority's refusal to fund a placement for him at the Home Farm Trust. This was an expensive resource, but one to which the local authority had made referrals in the past. Mark was able to show that it was a feature of his Down syndrome that a desire for certainty over his placement had become a psychological need. All the evidence then was that this was not only preferred accommodation, it was the only placement that could meet his psychological as well as his physical needs. An account of the case is given by Catriona Marchant in *Community Care*, 15 July 1993, p. 18.

Good practice would involve the provision of appropriate information about the range of accommodation on offer, with an opportunity to visit individual homes to compare their facilities and their philosophies of care. When residential care for older people is under discussion, social workers should be aware of the 'F' factor, where F stands for fear – the fears that older people have about remaining in their own home, whether that is fear of falling, fear of illness or fear of crime (DoH, 1995a). This fear is a reality for those oppressed by it and must be addressed; other means may exist to deal with that fear – occupational therapy assessment, for example, or the installation of an alarm system. Crisis admissions, which bypass or condense normal admission processes, should be carefully monitored, as should admissions precipitated by being in hospital. In one study, one-half of admissions to local authority homes were perceived as crisis admissions and six out of ten applicants and seven out of ten carers overall said that being in hospital had influenced the decision to apply (Neill et al., 1988). The introduction of reimbursement payments for delayed discharges (see Chapter 10) will exacerbate the conflicts between choice and the freeing up of acute hospital beds for older people in particular. Use of interim placements will increase and the direction on choice has been revised to enable interim placements to be made. The role of monitoring and review in such situations will be crucial, to support the fundamental principle of section 21 of the National Assistance Act 1948 that placements must meet people's assessed needs. Undoubtedly there remains a role for residential care within the spectrum of community care services.

For reasons to do with underfunding and stringent regulation, care capacity in residential settings for older people and people with physical disabilities shrank by 13,400 or 2.7 per cent of the total number of places in the 15 months to April 2003. Across all sectors, there were 74,000 fewer beds than in 1996 (Laing, 2003). An analysis of residential home closures between 1996 and 2001 found that the homes with a more intimate social environment were those most likely to have closed, thus reducing choice in a market which is more favourable to large corporate providers (Darton, 2004). The BMA expressed concern at its AGM in 2002 about the detrimental effects on patient care of the decline in the number of nursing and residential home beds, and believes that the solution is a better resourcing of community care and an end to the 'inequitable' (as it sees it) distinction between nursing and personal care and means-testing for those in need of long-term support. The demand for increased funding and the inadequacy of provision for vulnerable groups has been a recurrent theme since 1993. Residential care provision may be a symptom of the structured dependency of older people or it may simply be too tied up with bricks and mortar to be dismantled (Peace et al., 1997). The introduction of National Minimum Standards and the replacement of local authority registration and inspection units by monitoring from the CSCI has sought to introduce greater uniformity and predictability into residential care (see Chapter 6).

Concluding comments

Meeting the accommodation needs of users of social care services covers a wide spectrum of services from private and public housing to care home provision. There are difficult issues of capacity, most obviously encountered when dealing with homelessness or a contracting market for residential care. The social worker must not only work with housing as an external resource but has a significant role to play as a source of support for vulnerable tenants and people in transition from the community to more sheltered forms of accommodation, including residential care. This role is made more difficult by some conflicts of values within the system, for example pressures to respond to antisocial behaviour and to choose less expensive placements which arguably compromise the preferences of service users.

PAUSE AND REFLECT

1. Find out what types of accommodation are allocated by your local housing authority to people who are accepted as homeless.
2. Describe good practice in admission to residential care. What barriers exist to good practice and how can they be overcome?

CASE STUDY

Relocation

Mrs Maria Gawlinski, aged 85, is originally from Poland. Mrs Gawlinski's husband died two years ago and since then she has lived alone, with support from domiciliary services. Mrs Gawlinski is becoming increasingly confused and her only daughter, who lives 200 miles away, is concerned that her mother phones her anxiously several times a day to say that she is afraid of living alone. Mrs Gawlinski owns her own home.

What other housing options might be available to her, and what factors would need to be taken into account in considering a move from her own house.

FURTHER READING

Heywood, F., Oldman, C. and Means, R. (2002) *Housing and Home in Later Life*. Buckingham: Open University Press.
Examines the concept of home, when the relocation of older people is under discussion, and the range of accommodation and housing support services available to older people.

Joseph Rowntree Foundation (2002) *Britain's Housing in 2022*. York: Joseph Rowntree Foundation.
A projection of housing needs in 2022 recognising the links between tenure options and affordability.

CHAPTER 12

Working in Adult Services

Introduction

So far we have examined particular types of service provision in community care in the context of care management. But what impact have community care changes had on particular user groups such as older people, people with disabilities, mental health service users and users of specialist services such as substance misuse and HIV/AIDS services and asylum seekers? General trends may be discerned: the development of NSFs or National Minimum Standards guidance aimed at reducing local variations in service and prescribing particular models of service; the influence of user and carer involvement in the conceptualisation as well as planning of services; and the development of interagency cooperation at least in assessment and planning. Risk assessment and risk minimisation are, however, the current themes and the future development of systems, particularly in mental health, will see tensions between individual rights and public protection. Although organisational contexts and to some extent the knowledge base differentiate between different groups of service users, it is important to remember that most skills are generic and transferable and that distinctions between groups are social constructions rather than real differences.

KEY ROLE 6

Demonstrate professional competence in social work practice

The scope of adult services

Although the system of community care described in this book spans all adult user groups and is also applicable to children's services, the development of social work in the 1990s and beyond has seen a movement towards specialisation and away from genericism. In their examination of how community care is working out in practice, Lewis and Glennerster (1996) concluded that unified SSDs on the Seebohm model were becoming less sustainable. The publication in 2003 of the Green Paper *Every Child Matters* (DoH, 2003f) heralds a further step in this direction, with its emphasis on interagency and interprofessional working, the development of children's trusts and suggestions of new and separate qualifications for those working with children. The Children Act 2004 institutionalises the separation by requiring authorities to appoint directors of childrens services, most of whom will have an education rather than a social care background.

An assumption of unity may already be more apparent than real even within adult services. The term 'adult services' is a wide one, covering a range of different user groups with varying needs, interests and priorities. It is unlikely that any one model of service could be found that applies to all. Although all these groups will have been marginalised in the ways described in Chapter 1 through cultural stereotyping and service neglect, policy development post-community care has been somewhat different for each of them. In terms of theory and method, social work with these different groups will show distinctive differences. This chapter therefore traces the historical development of social work with different user groups, and analyses what community care has meant for each of them. Examples of innovation and good practice are given as appropriate.

Services for older people

Research into effective working with older people has shown the value of intensive involvement by qualified staff (Goldberg and Warburton, 1979), and work with older people in the community was the focus of the community care project in Kent (Davies and Challis, 1986), which became the blueprint for the development of care management as a general scheme. Thus, work with older people was at the forefront of community care development. Standardisation of older people's services across both the NHS and social services has been a more recent theme and is contained in the *National Service Framework for Older People* (DoH, 2001a). This NSF specifically addresses those conditions that are particularly significant for older people – stroke, falls and mental health problems in old age – but it also prioritises equitable treatment and quality of life issues for older people and their carers. It is based on eight standards:

1   Rooting out age discrimination by basing NHS services on clinical need and preventing SSDs from using age in their eligibility criteria to restrict access to services.
2   Person-centred care to be achieved through a single assessment process and integrated commissioning arrangements.
3   Access to a range of intermediate care services at home or in designated care settings to prevent unnecessary admission to hospital and provide effective rehabilitation.
4   General hospital care which respects privacy and dignity and which is appropriate and specialist.
5   Progress in reducing the incidence of stroke in the population and ensure prompt access to integrated stroke care services.
6   Objectives to reduce the number of falls that result in serious injury and ensure effective treatment and rehabilitation.
7   Access to integrated mental health services to ensure effective diagnosis, treatment and support, including support for carers. There is a focus on depression and dementia and recognition of the particular needs of older people from black and minority ethnic communities.
8   The promotion of health and active life expectancy in older people.

The emphasis on person-centred care, prevention and joint working is welcome. An Audit Commission report (2003a) found that older people too often received a disjointed approach when they needed help or advice. Building a common vision, values and approach was seen as more important than organisational arrangements, although the use of section 31 Health Act 1999 flexibilities has removed some structural barriers to closer working and changed thinking about planning and delivering services.

So how have older people themselves experienced service change? An SSI report (2002) found that the quality of services remains variable across the country. Ten years after the advent of community care, independent providers were not always regarded as real partners in service delivery and more action was required to address the needs of carers. Too many care plans were still resource-led, with eligibility criteria needing revision, but the area of most concern was the failure to review services. More positively, 70 per cent of service users were very satisfied with the service received and most assessments were based on a holistic approach. However, few councils were able to offer an intensive service to people from black and minority ethnic groups, and there was a shortage of services for people with mental health problems. Changing culture and practice, particularly in residential care, was also seen as more difficult to achieve than changing policies.

National implementation of the single assessment process has been much delayed. A number of models exist as assessment tools, all with the aim of cutting back on multiple assessments by different professionals, such as social workers, nurses, health visitors and housing officials, with the inevitable disparities in information held by each agency. All users/patients who request help will have a 'contact assessment', where basic personal information is collected and the nature of the presenting problem is explored to establish the presence of wider health or social care issues. Such an assessment may then lead on to either an overview assessment, an in-depth assessment or a comprehensive old age assessment. Thus the scale and depth of the assessment will vary depending on the needs presented, but its breadth will cover nine areas or 'domains' of need which impact on older people's independence, health and recovery or rehabilitation.

Most models of assessment are, however, based on medical models of diagnosis and treatment, posing a particular challenge to social care in clarifying and championing its particular value base (Guest, 2002). Guest is optimistic that this can be achieved and she sees the knowledge and experience of social care agencies in implementing care management as relevant to the principles of single assessment. There are others, however, who see social workers' use and experience of the care management process with older people as less positive. Gorman and Postle (2003), Lymbery (1998) and Richards (2000), for example, describe the difficulties that workers experience in trying to understand the needs of individual older people through a process dominated by agency agendas, complex legal and organisational frameworks and limited timescales that make older people passive recipients of an assessment, rather than active participants in decision-making. Workers also may experience what Postle (2002) sees as 'role ambiguity' in the conflict between work of increasing complexity and reductionist processes such as checklists, which a single assessment may fuel. New performance indicators from 2003–04 for adult social care will increase the pressure on throughput (see Chapter 12). This, combined with reimbursement policies on hospital discharge (see Chapter 9), will increase pressure for rapid assessments and early closure of cases, which will have a further impact on models of practice.

Older people with mental health problems

Services for older people with mental health problems pose particular challenges for both health and social care, in the light of demographic change. One-quarter of those over the age of 85 will develop dementia, with one-third of this group requiring constant care or supervision. In addition, depression is a common problem amongst older people, affecting between 10 and 16 per cent of those over 65 (Audit Commission, 2000). In the Audit Commission's research, specialist help for users and carers was found to be patchy and often uncoordinated, and although early diagnosis and treatment was seen to be important, a major difficulty was GPs' lack of training in the diagnosis and management of dementia. More than a decade after the early community care demonstration projects, the Audit Commission still needed to draw service planners' and practitioners' attention to the fact that people who would otherwise need residential care could live at home, if provided with flexible home-based care by joint health and social services teams. Research by Moriarty and Webb (1997) reinforces the message that the introduction of new or increased community services at assessment could delay the rate at which people with mild or moderate dementia were admitted to residential care. The conclusion to be drawn is that appropriate models of care management for people with dementia are those which can respond quickly to sudden changes and which target services to take account of the long-term and intensifying service needs for domiciliary, daycare and short-term care of this group.

   Despite the progress made between the Audit Commission's original report in 2000 and their update in 2002 (Audit Commission, 2002a), work is still needed in improving the process of reporting diagnosis and ensuring that older people and their carers are given access to relevant information about prognosis and services. As a resource for social workers and others engaged in the assessment of older people with mental health problems, SCIE (2002) has produced a practice guide which covers current policy and guidance, an overview of current practice, the Mental Health Act and older people and the needs of black and ethnic groups. Allen (2001) has also explored ways for staff in their day-to-day practice to consult people with dementia about their views and preferences, rather than them being seen as passive recipients of services.

Learning disability services

The history of services for people with learning disabilities is one of segregation and neglect (Means and Smith, 1994). The starting point for the change came as early as 1971 with the publication of a White Paper (DHSS/Welsh Office, 1971), which sought to establish a '20-year programme' for the resettlement of mentally handicapped people from the large institutions into the community. Progress was slow and the plan itself was overtaken by new concepts in working with the user group known by the late 1980s as 'people with learning disabilities' and more recently, in their own terms, as 'people with learning difficulties'. A more respectful terminology was accompanied by the development of the idea of 'ordinary living', which encompassed a range of accommodation, but mostly in ordinary housing and small group homes. Some specific resettlement projects were funded by the DSS and evaluated five years on by Cambridge et al. (1994) as part of a care in the community project. Interestingly, for this user group, community care proved to be more expensive than hospital care, even though little progress had been made in extending social networks and community participation. Social work input had also declined. Lack of employment and reliance on state benefits contributed to the marginalisation of residents (Cambridge et al., 1994).

The picture that comes across is of a lack of forward planning, in particular a failure to develop and provide services aggressively which would meet higher level needs such as the need for social stimulation, friendship and personal development. This narrowness of vision was echoed in Mencap's (1995, p. ii) survey of how community care was working at the level of individual assessments:

> Often assessments fall short of examining long-term needs and aspirations of people with learning disabilities and subsequent care packages severely limit the extent to which aspirations can be realised.

This approach was exacerbated by the use of checklist forms which concentrated on functional ability and the performance of activities of daily living, rather than people's own strengths and expectations.

The most important recent development was the publication of *Valuing People: A New Strategy for Learning Disability in the 21st Century* (DoH, 2000b). As the first White Paper on learning disability for 30 years, it reflects changes in values, services and approaches over that time. The White Paper highlights the fact that there are 1.2 million people with a mild or moderate learning disability in England. In addition, there are 120,000 adults and 25,000 people over pensionable age with a severe or profound learning difficulty, a significant increase on previous estimates. Working in partnership is to be a theme here for the development of services; learning disability partnership boards will have a key role in making sure that JIPs reflect the imperatives of the White Paper. The focus is person-centred planning (DoH, 2002f), with emphasis on the further development of care in the community, housing with support, advocacy and support for carers. Personal health action plans are seen as a way of improving health and access to services, and day services are to be refocused on links into employment. The emphasis is on choice, parity with other groups of disabled people, rights, independence and inclusion. There are also links with other modernising initiatives; priority for children with learning difficulties under Quality Protects, and links with Connexions for school-leavers facing transition.

So how has reality reflected the rhetoric of *Valuing People*? Research by Cope (2003) found that the fragmentation of organisational responsibilities meant that children with learning difficulties were often poorly equipped to make the transition to adult services. Also, more needed to be done to win the 'hearts and minds' of carers, if service users were to take advantage of new inclusive services. But, more fundamentally, good information and the support of an advocate, opportunities for increased choice and control over their lives was empty rhetoric for many people. There were some significant gaps in services for people from minority ethnic groups, and variations in access to health and *Supporting People* services. Also, the practice of closing cases, even for people with long-term needs when a package of care had been set up, was the norm; this meant that continuity was lost and families did not have a named social worker to refer to when circumstances changed. Again, there was a backlog of reviews, particularly for people in residential placements. The practice of social work with people with learning difficulties and their families appears to be struggling to meet the service aims and the value base of *Valuing People*.

Although guidance (DoH, 1999b) identified older people with a learning disability as a distinct service group, research undertaken by the SSI (1997) indicated that few authorities had fully developed plans to respond to changing life expectancy and increasing mental health needs with flexible daycare services and residential provision as a 'home for life'. Bigby (2004) concludes that social workers working with people with learning disabilities will need a wide range of knowledge and skills to span the developmental needs of individuals from adolescence through into old age. Grant (2001) also emphasises the importance of understanding life history and social and economic factors because older people with learning disabilities face a double jeopardy from disablism and ageism. The experiences of older carers are different too; carers who themselves are over the age of 60 comprise 44 per cent of carers of people with learning disabilities who live in the family home, and have accrued a lifetime of strengths and resilience which can be learned from to plan for the future as social networks shrink.

Further research by Cambridge et al. (2002) has assessed the impact of community care on the quality of life of people with learning disabilities by a follow-up study 12 years on from the original demonstration projects of the late 1980s. The study successfully involved service users in mapping their own social networks and classifying the nature of the contact and support they received, which was mainly with staff and other service users. The impression given is of a community within a community of former hospital patients, although 18 per cent of the original cohort were now living in accommodation with minimum staff support. In terms of planning for future costs, services that would be needed could not be predicted from the characteristics of users as measured in hospital 12 years earlier. Across the 12 sites surveyed, there was found to be wide variability in the organisation of care management and further difficulties of coordinating with care standards, personal care planning, the CPA and direct payments. These combined studies by Cambridge et al. in 1994 and 2002 present the largest longitudinal study of the deinstitutionalisation of learning disability services and the longest study of mental health services in the UK. As such, they demonstrate both the achievements and complexities of community care for an ageing population of care users.

Physical disability services

Pilling (1992) described the early British experience of care management for people with physical disabilities as an attempt to solve the problems of fragmentation and inflexibility for long-term user groups, according to models which either directly commission services (Davies and Challis, 1986), or act as service brokers on behalf of the user (Brandon and Towell, 1989). The disability movement would challenge this emphasis on the professional assessment of need, in arguments for citizenship and rights to service (Barnes et al., 2002). The social model of disability places independent living in the context of demands for human and civil rights, with users acting as their own care managers to access mainstream opportunities rather than segregated and stigmatised care (Kestenbaum, 1996). Thus the independent living movement challenges one of the basic assumptions of community care, that care itself is a worthwhile commodity to be bought and sold, or even to be provided informally, through what Morris (1994) calls 'the custodial nature of caring'.

Disabled people's early experience of community care and the social work service they had received was one of disappointment; many respondents to this SCOPE survey felt that whether or not they received services depended more on where they lived and whether there was sufficient money in the budget, rather than on their perceived needs (Lamb and Layzell, 1995). The introduction of charges for services and an inadequate level of service (particularly therapeutic health services such as physiotherapy and speech therapy) caused particular concern. Although the research was undertaken before the Carers Act introduced separate assessments for carers, two-thirds of carers interviewed felt that incorrect assumptions were being made about the help that was wanted, and that assessments did not take place regularly enough to take account of changing needs.

A report by the DoH (2003b) found that, although some progress was being made, many disabled people did not have the opportunities they seek to live independently and take control over their lives. The report found that:

- Home care was not sufficiently reliable or flexible
- Waiting times were unacceptably long for major adaptations
- Services for those with brain injury were not well enough developed
- Culturally sensitive services were not developed
- Disabled parents were often not effectively supported
- Day services needed reshaping to be more community-based
- Direct payments, although increasing, were not still seen as part of mainstream provision.

In demographic terms, identifying appropriate responses is a pressing issue. A report from the Prime Minister's Strategy Unit (2004) estimates that 20 per cent of the working age population is affected by disability, including long-term illness and mental health problems. Services are still seen as fragmented, and it is acknowledged that meaningful choice at key transition stages, such as entering employment and joining the housing market, is limited. The issues are formulated in terms of removing disabling barriers which give rise to reduced life choices for disabled people. These are seen as: discrimination (one in four disabled people have experienced hate crime or harassment); multiple disadvantage linked to class, ethnicity and age; lack of consultation; and poor access to buildings and transport.

The shortcomings of community care services for, respectively, younger people with physical disabilities (Fruin, 2000) and people with learning difficulties (Cope, 2003) have challenged the view that changes in policy will lead to changes on the ground. Fruin (2000), whilst acknowledging the progress that had been made towards independent living, found that the majority of young disabled people were still being offered services without any obvious consideration of whether they would promote independence. Progress towards implementing direct payments was described as 'disappointing' and joined-up approaches with health services were patchy in physical disability terms, although in learning disability services, joint commissioning and integrated teams had become the norm.

Social work practice with people with physical disabilities appears to have accepted rather than challenged structural and organisational limitations on a rights-based approach to assessment and service delivery. This view is reinforced by Rummery (2002), who looked at practice in two local authorities, covering both generic and specialist teams and hospital teams. The findings were analysed explicitly from a citizenship perspective in terms of whether or not the assessment process protects or enhances disabled people's status as competent members of society. Rummery found that access to assessment was treated as a privilege rather than a right, being subject to managerial, bureaucratic and professional gatekeeping. The competence of service users to define their own needs was variously undermined by professional reinterpretations and the prioritisation of family members' or carers' views. The workers most likely to take a civil rights approach in Rummery's view were those who worked in the specialist team for blind and partially sighted people. Evidence from respondents assessed in hospital and by other community teams, however, suggested that other pressures, such as the need to clear beds, save resources or limit the number of people receiving a full assessment, took precedence over treating applicants as co-citizens.

The NSF for long-term conditions (DoH, 2005) focuses on people with neurological conditions such as multiple sclerosis, but is also applicable to anyone with a long-term condition who is in need of health and social care services. The eleven quality requirements of the NSF include: person-centred care; early recognition; specialist acute management; a range of rehabilitation services; and support for family and carers in their own right. Like other NSFs, it is based on an expectation that health and social care will work together to anticipate and meet a range of needs in the community and hospital settings, with the full involvement of service users and an assumption that care and support will be provided for people to live independently wherever possible.

Parents with disabilities

Fair Access to Care Services (FACS) (DoH, 2002g) recognises that parents with disabilities may need support in their parenting role, and that it is appropriate for adult services to provide such support. A task force looking into support for disabled adults in their parenting role, however, received evidence that people with physical and sensory impairments, learning difficulties, mental health problems and long-term illness or HIV/AIDS experienced common barriers to receiving appropriate support, and that policies and services were often developed without consulting or involving disabled parents (Morris, 2003). Parents often find that they can get a response from services only in crisis situations and the inaccessibility of services can mean that children are asked to take on a young carer role. The task force found that this was a whole systems problem, with unequal access to health services and inadequate disability benefits compounding difficulties for parents with disabilities. The SSSI (2000) reported similar findings on the lack of coordination between services. Key messages for practitioners emphasise the requirement under the CA 1989 and Quality Protects to promote and strengthen family ties and deliver services in partnership. The SSI estimates the number of disabled parents to be between 1.2 and 4 million, with numbers thought to be increasing. Protocols for handling inter-team assessment work seem important here as well as multiagency services, and there is potential for the greater use of direct payments. Specific suggestions for effective practice are given (SSI, 2000):

- make certain you find out whether the disabled adult you are working with is a parent
- ensure that you know if a child with whom you are working has a disabled parent
- work with all the members of the family to empower disabled parents in their parenting role
- take account of the differing needs of all family members
- be aware of the impact of different disabilities on a person's ability to work in partnership with you.

People with multiple impairments

Developing adequate and effective services for people with multiple impairments is a major challenge for care management and highlights important issues in long-term work. An SSI (1993b) review of services for people with multiple impairments found that there was generally a focus on past events rather than future goals and on finding solutions to present difficulties rather than the enhancement of life potential. This had a particular impact on the conduct of reviews which were given low priority and lacked focus. If multidisciplinary working is absent, care plans tend to focus on the particular discipline or specialism of the practitioner. Contact with both health and social services may generally be perceived as irregular, infrequent and crisis-driven. Deterioration can happen quickly if support is withdrawn or not available. Continuity of service is therefore important, particularly to meet new developmental needs.

Mattingley (2002) identifies a skills gap for meaningful communication, particularly with people who have little or no speech, together with the frequent absence of effective advocacy services, neither of which are prioritised in FACS.

Holistic approaches like circles of support, which enable users, family members and staff to work together, are identified as an example of good practice in accessing and planning resources. In his research into the history and functioning of the Derbyshire Coalition for Independent Living, Priestley (2000) similarly locates the conflict which can arise between disabled people and local commissioning services within the discourses of personal tragedy, the impaired body and otherness, which lead to policy responses favouring the commodification of care, individualism and segregation. This is a direct challenge to policy-makers, including those who constructed the NSF for long-term conditions (DoH, 2005), who have traditionally focused on the effective provision of care, rather than a critical examination of its ideological significance.

Value-based tools do exist for working with people with profound and multiple impairments, most notably O'Brien and Lyle's (1987) 'five service principles' or 'accomplishments'. These are:

- *Common presence* – the sharing of the ordinary places that define community life
- *Choice* – the experience of autonomy in both small everyday matters and large life-defining matters
- *Competence* – the opportunity to perform functional and meaningful activities with whatever level or type of assistance required
- *Respect* – having a valued place among a network of people and valued roles in community life
- *Community participation* – the experience of being part of a growing network of personal relationships that include close friends.

In support of the five accomplishments, person-centred planning has been adopted as a method of understanding and enhancing the aspirations of people living in a range of settings, whether in the community or elsewhere (O'Brien and O'Brien, 2000). Person-centred planning has emerged as an ethical method of intervention, based on developmental principles, that enlists people with disabilities and their families and supporters in seeing people first rather than relating to diagnostic labels. It asks 'what has to change to make the person's dream come true'? Person-centred planning thus acts as a microcosm for community care practice more generally by bringing people together into 'communities of practice', bound together by expertise as practitioners, service users or carers, in a joint enterprise. It feeds into the process of care management by identifying personal preferences and needs but, unlike care management, has no statutory constraints or limitations imposed by eligibility criteria or charging regimes (DoH, 2002f).

Sensory impairments

Social work services for people who are blind or deaf are often separated from the mainstream. The SSI (1997b) found that sensory impairment workers generally stood outside care management structures and were organisationally isolated. Research by Lovelock et al. (1995) into the social support needs of visually impaired people, however, emphasised the 'generic' as well as the 'specialist' understanding required particularly in the case of older people with sight-related needs who sought assessment for services. The British Deaf Association's (1996) report concluded that deaf people's effective participation in local services was dependent upon proactive measures which included training in skill-building, assertiveness and confidence-raising. Deaf clubs are an important cultural focus, and the employment of deaf workers or the use of deaf facilitators is an indicator that formal agencies are approachable.

Services for people who are deafblind have received particular attention. Guidance (DoH, 2001l) notes that at least 40 people per 100,000 are deafblind and many are not known to their local services authority. Principles for the appropriate assessment and provision of services to deafblind people are set out:

- assessments should be carried out by a specifically trained person/team
- mainstream services may not be appropriate for those with a dual impairment
- specifically trained one-to-one support workers may be needed
- information should be provided in formats and by methods that are accessible to deafblind people.

Cultural issues therefore dictate the model of service that is appropriate for this user group.

Transition services

The interface between child and adult services is not always smooth so as to facilitate transitions and ensure a seamless service for users (Hirst and Baldwin, 1994; SSI 1996b). Workshops organised nationally by the SSI to look at transition services produced both a management and a user agenda (SSI/DoH, 1996). The management agenda was to minimise disparity in services, but the user agenda was for disability equality training within agencies to promote understanding of the potentially conflicting views of young people and their parents. Users thus emphasise the importance of having a forum for discussion with assessors and service providers and for self-advocacy services. They also recognise the importance of traditional social work skills in negotiation and mediation within families.

The legislative framework for promoting smooth transitions for school-leavers is in principle already in place. Sections 5 and 6 of the Disabled Persons Act 1986 require schools to consult with SSDs when children who are statemented with special educational needs (SEN) reach the first annual review after their fourteenth birthday. This enables the SSD to identify which of those children it will regard as 'disabled' within the meaning of section 29 of the National Assistance Act 1948 for whom further assessment will be necessary. The requirements of the Disability Discrimination Act 1996 have also been brought into education through the Special Educational Needs and Disability Act 2001 which extends to colleges and universities as well as schools. A new code of practice accompanying the Act places greater emphasis on parental involvement, forward planning and dispute resolution; however, SEN services are under increasing pressure as the number of children with a statement has risen by 35 per cent since 1992 (Audit Commission, 2000).

Transition planning has been observed to be particularly difficult to get right for young people in out of county residential school placements (Abbott et al., 2001) and referral forms designed with older people in mind may not reflect younger people's background and aspirations (SSI/DoH, 1996). Despite a clear legislative and regulatory framework, research continues to show that transition planning is often characterised by poor liaison between different agencies and professionals, a failure to involve young people and a lack of recognition of the importance of family life (Morris, 2003). In one study, a survey of 283 families, a third of young people with learning difficulties did not have a transition plan at all (Heslop et al., 2001). Clearly, there is still much progress to be made in bridging the divide between children's and adult services. Morris (2002) identifies personal advisers in the Connexions service and young persons' advisers under the Children (Leaving Care) Act as having an important role to play in improving transition planning. *Valuing People* (DoH, 2000b) also emphasises planning for transition on a multiagency basis; and the extension of direct payments to disabled 16–17-year-olds by the Carers and Disabled Children Act 2000 will enable young people to plan their future independently of traditional services.

Mental health services

Services for people with mental health problems reflect the two policy strands of closure of the large institutions and the development of services for people in the community. Goodwin (1989) examines the reasons behind the policy of deinstitutionalisation after 1954, and observes a mixture of social democratic egalitarianism and pragmatism in the development of smaller, community-based psychiatric units, a growth in the number of community mental health nurses (CMHNs) and the development of domiciliary and daycare services. The 'pharmacological revolution', and especially the development of psychotropic drugs, has enabled people to be given medication to assist them to live in the community when previously they would have been detained in hospital (Jones, 1993). Care in hospital has thus become only one of a range of services available for people who are mentally ill. Most people will be treated by their GP and may in fact never be referred to specialist psychiatric services. Care in the community is seen as a cheaper option at a time of financial pressure, as well as legitimising the intrusive nature of some psychiatric services by locating them in a normal environment (Goodwin, 1989). Of more general concern is insufficient support for the concept of care and treatment as a right, and the creation of an accepting and enabling community with an active approach to rehabilitation and support (Bennett and Morris, 1983).

The *Mental Health National Service Framework* was published in 1999 (DoH, 1999), the second NSF to be created. It sets out national standards for mental healthcare for people of working age and takes the form of a ten-year plan to be implemented in stages through local implementation teams in health and social care communities. The National Institute for Mental Health (NIMHE) has also been set up originally within the Modernisation Agency at the Department of

Health to improve outcomes for people using mental health services. Finally, the draft Mental Health Bill 2004 develops the policy set out in the 2000 White Paper (DoH, 2000e). Mental health is thus actively on the policy agenda, not only for systems change, but also for new ways of collaborative working, some of which may cut across existing professional boundaries and may challenge the value base of those working in mental health services.

The NSF for mental health is based around seven standards:

1   Mental health promotion, the combating of discrimination and promotion of social inclusion.
2   Access to the identification, assessment and treatment of common mental health problems within primary care, including referral to specialist services if required.
3   24-hour access to local services and NHS Direct.
4   Risk minimisation and crisis prevention for patients on the care programme approach, including care plans.
5   Timely access to an appropriate hospital bed or alternative which is in the least restrictive environment, and a copy of the written aftercare plan.
6   Annual assessment of carers' needs and a written care plan.
7   Action necessary to reduce suicide.

Major investment is being made in new modes of service delivery: crisis resolution, or home treatment on a 24-hour basis; assertive outreach to improve engagement with people with multiple and complex needs; and early intervention in psychosis for younger people aged up to the age of 35. This is clearly a challenging agenda for both health and social care. The SSI report (2002a) identified strengths and weakness in the existing system from a social care perspective. It found that services were starting from a low baseline in terms of quality and availability, especially 'after hours' services. Areas particularly in need of development were effective working with children's services and meeting the needs of black and minority ethnic communities (DoH, 2003a). There were also continuing shortcomings in the CPA as a whole system approach to care, rather than as a mechanism for managing reviews.

The *Mental Health Policy Implementation Guide* (DoH, 2002b) commends community mental health teams (CMHTs) as an appropriate vehicle for the function of collaboration between key stakeholders. The service is designed for two groups of users: a majority who will have time-limited disorders and who will be referred back to their GPs after five or six contacts; and a minority who will remain with the team for ongoing treatment, care and monitoring for periods of several years. An integrated model of the CPA is expected to be applied across health and social care, instead of a dual system. This in itself will require singly managed teams, using one set of client records. A CMHT requires the skills of nursing, social work, psychology and medicine to carry out the full range of interventions from psychological therapies to physical healthcare, emotional and carer support, help in accessing work and education, the basics of daily living, treatment of substance abuse and relapse prevention. Through coordinating with other systems, CMHTs thus provide a discrete and internally coherent system for working with mental disorder, facilitating referrals and offering specialist advice. At the same time, there is a focus on privacy and dignity in inpatient care (DoH, 2002c) and support for carers (DoH, 2002d).

Recent policy changes such as the NSF have sought to combine organisational efficiency with person-centred approaches and there have been considerable practice changes. The strengths perspective, which has been particularly influential in training, seeks to depathologise the individual through empower-ment, resilience and membership (Saleeby, 2002). It challenges the distance, power inequality, control and manipulation that can mark the relationship between helpers and helped. The focus on building on strengths, coupled with a 'right to care' and support for families and communities, affirms the core values of social work and provides 'a distinctive lens for examining the world of practice' (Saleeby, 2002 p. 20). It is an approach which has also been advocated for clients with substance misuse problems, where it has been shown to have an impact on retention in treatment, drug use severity and involvement in the criminal justice system (Rapp, 2002; DoH/NAT, 2003). There are parallels between Rapp's approach and care management, insofar as the case manager becomes a service broker in the search for resources identified by the client as promoting their individual treatment plan; a 'welcome relief' to clients who typically have been involved with numerous, disparate resources at any one time (Rapp, 2002, p. 141).

In this context, *The Journey to Recovery: The Government's Vision for Mental Healthcare* (DoH, 2001e) provides an overview of policies adopted by government to improve mental health services for people of working age and change the focus from chronicity to recovery. The guiding principles for the future development of this policy are stated to be:

- a commitment to recovery
- the use of community resources
- claiming citizenship
- changing public perceptions.

Although the concept of recovery is new in the guidance, its emphasis on individual control and the person's ownership of their mental illness can be identified within the central principles of long-established self-help organisations (Turner-Crowson and Wallcraft, 2002). It is also linked with personal narrative approaches to understanding the needs of mental health service users as opposed to the medically driven agendas of traditional mental health services. From a users' perspective, MIND's (2001) report was based on the charity's largest ever survey of people with mental health problems, and explores their understanding of recovery and the social and emotional factors that help them in this process (Warren, 2003).

The future development of the mental health workforce is explored by the Department of Health (2004e) in terms of 'the ten essential shared capabilities' which cut across, but do not replace professional boundaries and National Occupational Standards. Essential shared capabilities provide the mental health-specific context and achievements for education, training and continuing professional development at pre-registration/qualification stage. They are overtly value-based and comprise:

- Working in partnership
- Respecting diversity
- Practising ethically
- Challenging inequality
- Promoting recovery
- Identifying people's needs and strengths
- Providing service user-centred care
- Making a difference
- Promoting safety and positive risk-taking
- Personal development and learning.

This emphasis on shared capabilities is increasingly important in the development of CMHTs and in the context of proposals to introduce approved mental health professionals from a range of backgrounds to replace approved social workers under the Mental Health Act.

Substance misuse

Before the implementation of the NHSCCA 1990, services for substance misuse (chiefly drug and alcohol services) consisted mainly of residential detoxification and rehabilitation funded through social security payments, and hospital treatment as part of the NHS (SSI, 1994). The decision to include drug and alcohol misuse services within the remit of the NHSCCA 1990, and transfer funding by this means, was intended to give local authorities scope to commission a comprehensive needs-led network of services. Expertise, however, continues to be located primarily in healthcare services and the voluntary sector.

Substance misuse has been recognised (DoH, 1990) as a significant public health problem associated with social problems such as offending, homelessness, unemployment, family breakdown, domestic violence and child abuse. There are, however, inherent difficulties in the commissioning of substance misuse services (SSI, 1994), because of:

- stigma
- the absence of accurate prevalence data, due particularly to a reluctance to disclose the illegality of drug use
- the aetiology of substance misuse which may make intervention dependent upon readiness to change
- delay in service response to changing patterns of misuse.

This is a complex service area, at an early stage of development, in which social services agencies are trying to define and establish their roles and place themselves more at the centre of service planning and development. The expectation is that people who misuse alcohol and drugs should be receiving services of the same standard as other adults accessed through the framework of community care in collaboration with other community care services and other agencies.

The most recent policy guidance on substance misuse is contained in the government's ten-year drugs strategy (Home Office, 1998). This focuses on four key areas: prevention strategies with younger people; community protection; treatment; and limiting availability. Overall responsibility lies with the Drugs

Strategy Directorate of the Home Office. Relevant targets are an increase in the participation of problem drug users in treatment programmes by 50 per cent in 2004, and 100 per cent in 2008, and (within the NHS plan) to reduce levels of drug-related deaths by 20 per cent by 2004. Delivery of the treatment target is overseen by the National Treatment Agency (NTA) for substance misuse, set up in 2001 as a special health authority. Local delivery of the drug strategy is planned and coordinated by drug action teams.

Models of Care for the Treatment of Adult Drug Misusers (DoH/NTA, 2003) sets out a national framework for the commissioning of an integrated treatment system for drug misuse and serves as a framework for further guidance on alcohol misuse. The national agenda to improve the quality and capacity of drug treatment services has been influenced by wider developments for improving health and social services in general, such as the need to reduce waiting times for treatment and develop consistent, high-quality care centred on patients. It highlights partnerships between health and social services with the voluntary and independent sectors. The guidance responds to the 2003 Audit Commission report, which found that many areas of the county had limited drug treatment options, with a lack of planning and coordination. Particularly neglected groups were crack misusers, black and minority ethnic drug misusers and services for women and those leaving prison. *Models of Care*, however, reiterates the priority of harm-minimising, rather than abstinence. The commissioning of services through integrated care pathways is based on a four-tier framework, designed (as with other NSFs) to provide equitable access to drug treatment services across the country, according to an increasing severity of need.

The model of care management preferred in the guidance is modelled on the CPA for mental health service users, comprising standard care coordination and enhanced care coordination for those with complex needs. The processes of care planning, monitoring and review are set out in the guidance as requirements that commissioners should ensure are met, and it is anticipated (DoH/NTA, 2003, para. 7.1) that care planning and care coordination should be undertaken by a 'range of professionals'.

Considerable overlap exists between individual service users' needs. A dual diagnosis of mental disorder and substance misuse is one of the most common interactions, and the DoH (2002b) has produced a good practice guide in this area. CMHTs typically report (p. 7) that 8–15 per cent of their clients have a dual diagnosis. Correlations in the criminal justice system are even higher, with 79 per cent of male remand prisoners who were drug-dependent having two or more additional mental disorders (p. 8). Substance misuse is also associated with increased rates of violence and suicidal behaviour (p. 9). This is not 'new work' for either set of agencies, but is about achieving a more integrated and effective framework covering mental health, better diagnosis and training and utilisation of the CPA for long-term engagement.

HIV/AIDS

People with HIV/AIDS present significant challenges to both social and healthcare agencies because of their complex and often rapidly changing needs, which demand close collaboration between agencies to ensure that these are met in a timely and appropriate manner (DoH, 1994a). In contrast with services for substance misusers, the Department of Health's (1994a) study of community care implementation revealed a commitment to joint planning, significant involvement of voluntary agencies and a profile within community care plans as a feature of community care for people with HIV/AIDS.

According to the UK HIV and AIDS statistics summary (DoH, 2003e), at the end of 2003, there were approximately 41,200 people living with HIV/AIDS in the UK, about 30 per cent of whom were undiagnosed. A report commissioned by the National Aids Trust recommended the mainstreaming of HIV services into a wider sexual health strategy, taking a 'communities at risk' focus, rather than a narrow disease focus (Bonell, 2000). The report also explores the non-health-based aspects of HIV/AIDS care such as mental health, employment and benefits, family support and HIV-related discrimination. Recommended clinical standards for NHS HIV services (Medical Foundation for AIDS and Sexual Health, 2003; DoH, 2003c) fit into *The National Strategy for Sexual Health and HIV* (DoH, 2001c), to develop a patient-centred care pathway and build on the policy aims of organisations active in the field. A series of standards is outlined, covering both primary and secondary care, with links to other government initiatives.

It is acknowledged, within the framework, that social needs may predominate for people with HIV, particularly those with families. Guidance (DoH, 2003h) advises local authorities in devising their HIV social care plans to take into account the need for comprehensive population needs assessment, being especially aware of the needs of minority groups, including asylum seekers, and effective joint arrangements with housing, health commissioners and providers, voluntary and independent providers and service users and carers. In addition, direct payments may be considered to be particularly suitable for people whose needs are complex and fast changing, and services should also be integrated with children and families' services and services for people with drug related problems. The value of social interventions is described in research by White and Cant (2003), in which they explore the positive links between social support and the health and well-being of a group of HIV-positive gay men. Using social network analysis, they describe patterns of emotional and practical support within a social rather than a medical model of care.

Asylum seekers

Adult asylum seekers, both in their own right and as heads of families, may present as 'in need of community care services', thus triggering the assessment duty of the local authority. The law relating to asylum seekers and other persons subject to immigration control is complex and fast moving. Its ideological roots are discernable in terms of protecting boundaries, rationing welfare support and negotiating the balance between central government and local administrations. The Immigration and Asylum Act 1999 removed the right of asylum seekers to access mainstream welfare benefits, public housing and most forms of local authority assistance. The National Asylum Support Service (NASS) is now responsible for supporting destitute asylum seekers in the UK. Even that support, based as it is on dispersal for accommodation and means-tested support at below poverty levels, is denied to those who have not claimed asylum 'as soon as reasonably practicable', normally at the port of arrival in the UK. This provision, the controversial section 55 of the Nationality, Immigration and Asylum Act 2003, has been successfully challenged in the Court of Appeal, to the extent that destitute asylum seekers left without basic amenities were seen to be subject to cruel, inhuman and degrading treatment in breach of Article 3 of the European Convention on Human Rights. The Refugee Council report (2004) showed that of 130 organisations working with asylum seekers, 74 per cent had seen clients forced to sleep rough, go hungry or survive without basic essentials such as clothes and toiletries. Asylum seekers who are in need of care and attention because of age or disability are entitled to accommodation under section 21 of the National Assistance Act 1948, and young people, including unaccompanied minors who were formerly looked after children, will receive continuing support under the Children (Leaving Care) Act 2000.

Resettlement practice in relation to asylum seekers and refugees needs simultaneously to focus on healthcare needs, cultural and economic needs, psychosocial needs and the enhancement of resilience in order to meet developmental opportunities in the new environment (Kohli and Mather, 2003). The limitation of welfare assistance, the dispersal policy of the NASS away from community support and the continuing pressure of racism and xenophobia militate against successful resolutions. This aspect of community care is thus effectively supervised by local communities and non-funded voluntary groups dealing with considerable deprivation, reactive mental health needs and problems of settlement and relocation.

This theoretical basis of social work with asylum seekers and other immigrant groups has been considered by Hayes and Humphries (2004). They point to the social construction of a separate and inferior welfare system for such groups and see social workers as having been compliant in this, through their role in gatekeeping resources rather than meeting need. Social workers caught up in a familiar conflict between care and control have been instrumental in adapting media stereotypes of deserving and undeserving applicants for asylum. Ironically:

> the factors social workers would consider significant in assessing risk are almost identical to the conditions we are placing asylum seekers in, for example, extreme poverty, isolation, separation, negative labelling, scapegoating and hostility. (Hayes and Humphries, 2004, p. 220)

Yet despite these structural barriers, Kohli and Mather (2003) provide a more positive opportunity for practice with asylum seekers based on a strengths perspective. Blackwell (1997) sees the appropriate role for a worker as being that of 'witness' to trauma, through the process of holding and containing, and not necessarily that of a rescuer, particularly when questioning can be mistaken for interrogation. Helping people to make sense of what happened in the past and providing a secure base from which they can progress are central to the task of supporting the psychological needs of asylum seekers, even in the absence of physical resources (Kohli and Mather, 2003).

Concluding comments

This chapter has shown the wide variations in people who may call on social workers to respond to their needs in a community care context. The knowledge base is wide and has extended, with developments in legislation and policy which have meant that community care services have become relevant to more diverse groups of people. Some of the themes explored in earlier chapters, such as the relationship between social care and healthcare and housing, are played out in practice with these particular user groups. Methods of working may be prescribed by NSFs which set standards against which local services will be evaluated, but there are still some basic, unresolved tensions between the fundamental issues of care and control, particularly in mental health services, and now in relation to working with asylum seekers. But despite the focus on frameworks for service, a commitment to therapeutic work remains a part of the social work task. Person-centred planning focuses on individual aspirations and strengths, and challenges formal services and the community to respond to these expressed needs. Social work with older people also recognises the importance of life review and narrative in understanding and therefore planning alongside people. Recognising that individuals have different identities as service users requires us to acknowledge individuals' need to care for others whether as parents or supporters. Community care practice must involve all these groups as architects of service provision and interpreters of their own strengths and futures.

PAUSE AND REFLECT

Examine provision locally for any adult user group. To what extent do services offer opportunities for:

- a smooth transition from children's services to adult services
- support to people who are parents
- support to people who have long-term physical conditions.

CASE STUDY

Criminal justice and community care

Ronald Victor is a 45-year-old man with a long history of drug and alcohol misuse. He has previous convictions and is currently nearing the end of a 12-month prison sentence imposed for a number of public order offences and an assault on a police officer. His physical and mental health are both impaired and he is of no fixed abode.

If you were Ronald's probation officer, what sort of services might you be considering for Ronald and what use might you make of community care legislation?

FURTHER READING

DoH (2000) *Valuing People: A New Strategy for Learning Disability for the 21st Century.* London: Stationery Office.
The first White Paper on learning disability for 30 years, it shows how attitudes have changed over time and what remains to be done.

Royal Commission on Long Term Care (1999) *With Respect to Old Age.* London: Stationery Office.
Comprehensive review of the needs of older people, demographic changes and service options for health and social care.

SSI (2002) *Modernising Mental Health Services.* London: Stationery Office.
Reviews recent changes in mental health policy and evaluates their impact on actual service delivery.

Conclusion

Community care, as it has developed historically, cannot be described in terms of one system, despite common ideological roots and a single legislative framework. The development of services for older people, those with mental health problems, those with disabilities and other groups has been influenced by historical antecedents, demographic issues and the diverse concerns of professionals and service users. The knowledge base of community care has become so large that a return from specialisation to genericism in the delivery of services is probably unrealistic. However, the major infrastructure issues have commonalties. The provision of social care cannot be isolated from healthcare, housing and financial support. In all these areas, major change has taken place, emphasising both the split between purchasers and providers of services and, in its wake, the mixed economy of public and independent sector provision. Support from informal carers has been a basic tenet on which community care has been built. Chiefly, however, this has been provided by families rather than communities, meaning that individualism has been the basic model of service provision in community care.

What is controversial is the extent to which community care has changed not only the context and style but also the meaning of social work practice. By emphasising efficiency in the allocation of resources and the rationality of competition, business skills have been incorporated into the job that social workers do. Providing support and advocacy for vulnerable and disadvantaged people will necessarily involve values and choices which fit uneasily into this framework. Community care is a system based on needs, not rights. The social worker's role in assessing need means that he or she acts as a gatekeeper for potential users of services. How many people are allowed to enter the system and according to what criteria will vary in relation to the amount of resources the agency has at its disposal, its policy decisions concerning competing demands on those resources and its interpretation of its legal obligations towards different individuals and groups. Arguably, this compromises professionalism by the constraints that it imposes on the breadth of an assessment or the range of choices that can subsequently be offered. Tensions may exist between economic and social objectives, managing the budget and advocacy for the best deal possible for an individual who is seeking a service.

These sorts of dilemma mean that social work cannot be atheoretical. Community care policy is based on a consensus model of society within which change is seen as incremental and based on rational principles. This is overlaid by a belief in personal responsibility and family values. Thus the means-testing of payment for services and the emphasis on informal, or family-based, care may be seen to reflect a system based on unequal opportunities and traditional roles. The role of the social worker may be seen as ameliorating the harshness of economic forces with respect to some groups or individuals seen as deserving or unfortunate. Radical perspectives would, by contrast, emphasise the importance of challenging structural inequalities rather than working within them. Anti-oppressive practice highlights structural and individual aspects of oppression based on race, gender, sexuality, disability and social class. The theoretical orientation of the worker will in turn determine the method of intervention which is favoured as well as the outcome that is sought. Despite its prescribed emphasis on procedures and process, the need for reflective and analytical practice is thus enhanced rather than undermined by community care.

At the structural level, the strength of community care has been that it has allowed strategic planning to take place, often on an interagency basis. The requirements that agencies should produce service delivery plans has required them to be explicit about what services they can provide, what services are the responsibility of other agencies and their criteria for accessing services according to different levels of need. This in turn has made the whole administrative decision-making process more transparent and therefore more open to challenge. There have, however, been lost opportunities. Community social work has not been much developed, except through the limited introduction of action zones targeted at education or healthcare needs. Nor has anti-oppressive practice developed to the point where it has significantly enhanced community support. Social work under community care has thus continued to focus on the specific needs of individuals, albeit in a family and community context. This has in turn meant that the traditional methods and values of social casework have retained a continuing validity within community care, but it has also meant that care *by* the community has been less well developed than care *in* the community.

Achieving a consensus between agencies, and between agencies and service users, on the proper definition of need has been more controversial. An assessment of need is the gateway to service provision, but 'need' itself is a term with a shifting meaning according to changing political and economic circumstances. Service planning must also be responsive to needs which may not previously have been well articulated. The needs of carers, for example, have only recently found legislative expression in the Carers and Disabled Children Act 2000, which gives those who provide a substantial amount of care on a regular basis a right to an assessment of their needs separate from that of the service user. The appropriateness of traditional service provision also needs to be evaluated. Services for black communities, for example, require significant reappraisal. The disability movement has also raised basic issues about the worthwhileness of care as a commodity in its own right. In the field of housing in particular, the importance of fine-tuning mainstream services as well as making specialist provision have emphasised the 'ordinary life' principles of community care as integration within living and working communities. In a fundamental sense, this is what community care was intended to achieve: the ending of separate and segregated provision, and the enhancement instead of people's ability to live and develop within their own communities.

Ensuring a firm value base for the development of social work within community care is absolutely fundamental. Social workers, especially in the role of care manager, will be constrained by agency policies and procedures and necessarily so, but this does not absolve them from the professional imperative to respect the lifestyles and choices of the people with whom they work. Arguably, respecting difference can be facilitated within the system of community care. It may be argued that the emphasis on due process within a bureaucratic model enables advocacy to flourish and unarticulated value positions in service provision to be challenged. Moves towards proceduralism also challenge social workers to analyse their practice more precisely. The emphasis on monitoring and review within care management requires the criteria for progress or success to be fixed more clearly at the assessment stage. There is thus less scope for ill-focused, and arguably oppressive, intervention when the mandate for involvement has to be agreed by all concerned at the outset. Agreeing and delivering on such a mandate also requires basic and enduring social work skills in communication, assessment, negotiation and reflection. The conclusion to be drawn is that social work per se continues to have a role within community care, in terms of the knowledge, skills and values that it brings to the task.

The goals of community care were explicitly to restore and maintain independence by enabling people to live in the community, promote individual choice and self-determination, clarify the responsibility of agencies and make practical support for carers a high priority. The White Paper (1989b) which propounded these principles was subtitled *Community Care in the Next Decade and Beyond*. The agenda was undoubtedly an ambitious one, wide ranging in its scope and fundamental to the very functioning of a welfare state. It would be extraordinary if the ramifications of such an agenda for community care and social work could be fully explored within the space of one decade. The Blair government of 1997 onwards had the task of developing its own interpretation of community care and reflecting critically on the system it inherited. Its emphasis is on social inclusion and a recognition that all people face personal and family crises to which social services should be able to respond effectively. All people therefore will have an interest in efficient and well coordinated services. The White Paper *Modernising Social Services* (DoH, 1998a) emphasises three things: promoting independence; improving protection; and raising standards. The provision of social care services is seen not just as a safety net for the minority but a guarantee of quality for the majority. Improving joint working between health and social services through partnership and ensuring greater consistency in the availability and cost of services in different parts of the country through the centralising tendency of policy guidance are clearly stated policy aims. A better qualified workforce, which will in turn be monitored through clearer and more objective inspection arrangements, is seen as central to an improvement in standards. Client satisfaction surveys are also seen as important in the development of user-centred services. All these ideas are central tenets of community care policy presented in social democratic rather than New Right terms. There is less emphasis on market forces, but the role of the independent sector continues to be emphasised. A feature of the system is greater control by central government of local spending priorities, through the use of special and specific grants, and the evaluation of service effectiveness against preset targets by arm's-length inspection bodies. Regulation has thus replaced crude notions of market competition as a monitor of quality.

For the social work practitioner, the impact of *Modernising Social Services* is a greater emphasis on professional and public accountability. Workforce standards will be monitored by the General Social Care Council, with responsibility not only for social workers but for the million or more other staff who constitute the social care workforce. Regulation of care standards is taken away from local control and invested in the national Commission for Social Care Inspection which will regulate not only residential care but domiciliary care and also local authority services, according to national standards. The protection of vulnerable children and adults from abuse and neglect has received further consideration; for children this will also include developing life chances and specifically improving transitions from care to independent adult life. Overall, the emphasis will be on greater clarity and consistency in service provision, supporting independence – including an expansion of direct payments – and meeting targets for efficiency improvements.

The New Right faith in market competition has been replaced by a legislative mandate in some cases to cooperate. So health and social care are required to make use of the Health Act flexibilities in order to break down barriers between the two organisations. The internal market within the NHS has also been dismantled in favour of a primary care-led system and encouragement of autonomy as a reward for meeting targets. In some cases, new players have been brought onto the scene to undertake the task of coordination; examples are *Supporting People* teams in housing and the Connexions service for young people in education. The views of service users and carers are formally represented in the planning and delivery of services and in reviews. Social exclusion has been tackled, not so much by the development of notions of community responsibility but by policies on employment and welfare designed to move minority groups into the mainstream. NSFs have been designed to minimise differences in the type and quality of service available in different localities and outcome measures have increasingly been used to evaluate the effectiveness of services. The movement away from directly provided services has continued but eligibility for service is increasingly based on risk rather than need. This rationing of services and the development of managerialism has had the effect of highlighting conflicts between the demands of the agency for rapid and consistent decision-making and considered professional discretion. With adult services and children's services developing to a large extent independently of each other even at the level of central government, the coherence of social work training is in jeopardy. This is despite the fact that the key roles which social care workers perform are recognisable and attainable across all types of agency and in all settings.

In April 2004, the government stated its intention to parallel the Green Paper *Every Child Matters* (DoH, 2003f) with a vision and framework for the future of adult social care (DoH, 2004). The launch of a consultation on the context of the proposed statement was prefaced by a statement from the responsible minister that this new vision should put the person needing support at its centre, 'rather than the institutions providing that support'. It should be a vision that 'promotes inclusion and diversity and supports people in their choices and aspirations rather than "cares" for them once all choice and hope is gone' (DoH, 2004). The emphasis is placed on services which are:

- *Person-centred* – tailored to the individual's circumstances and enabling people to fulfil their potential
- *Proactive* – intervening in time to prevent problems and help people to maintain their independence
- *Seamless* – working with partner agencies and professionals to remove gaps and improve coordination and accessibility.

It is likely that the framework for adult social services will include sections on:

- What service users and carers want from services
- The values and vision that should underpin provision and practice
- The legislative and policy framework for social care and links to policies in related areas like public health, the NHS, employment and training
- The changing role of local authorities in assessing the needs of service users, commissioning services and promoting well-being
- New requirements and expectations of the social care workforce
- Arrangements for regulation and performance management.

Further developments in the organisation of the NHS are also anticipated. *The NHS Improvement Plan* (DoH, 2004a) sets out the priorities of the NHS until 2008 and builds on the NHS plan of July 2000. The reforms of 2000 are presented as having produced a fairer, better-resourced system; the next stage is a drive for responsive, convenient and personalised services, with an emphasis on choice in hospital care and support in the community for people with long-term conditions, as well as a focus on prevention. This is the next stage in the development of community care. PCTs will control 80 per cent of NHS budgets and will be able to commission services from treatment centres, located in the independent sector, as well as from foundation trusts. This will expand capacity and choice and further limit waiting times. A mixed economy of care, based on free-market principles of choice, will be encouraged for health, as it has been for social care.

Generally, the focus has shifted from targeting resources on those most in need or at risk towards prevention and social inclusion. Discussion of the values on which policy and practice should be based has become more overt. One example of this is the person-centred approach taken by *Valuing People* (DoH, 2000b) towards people with learning difficulties; another is the desire to 'invert the triangle of care' (ADSS/LGA, 2003) for older people to confront ageism and recognise the vital role that older people play in society. Cooperation between health and social care is seen as critical, but so too is the extension of universal services including transport and lifelong learning. There has been an attempt to move ideologically away from welfare towards a citizenship agenda. This movement has been reflected in the title of the Green Paper on adult social care: *Independence, Well-being and Choice* (DoH, 2005a). The Green Paper talks about harnessing the capacity of communities under a director of adult services within local authorities, but with a brief wider than social care. The voluntary and community sector will be encouraged to expand in order to develop new service models based on strategic needs assessments, including the wider use of direct payments and individual budgets, common assessment tools (with greater use of self-assessment), extra care housing and assistive technology. The social work role would be that of 'navigator', akin to a service broker, rather than a care manager. The real control would then be in the hands of individuals and communities, with specialist staff focusing on complex needs. Care *in* the community would then become care *by* the community, with opportunities for all people to play a part.

PAUSE AND REFLECT

Consider the extent to which interagency and partnership working and increased regulation has changed the social worker's role. Looking at the six key roles within the National Occupational Standards, reflect on the implications of these changes for your future career in social work, in terms of the settings within which you will work and the job you will do.

CASE STUDY

Adult and children's services

Shelley Todd is 28 years old and a long-standing user of mental health services; she also takes street drugs and has a number of convictions relating to her drug use. She is a single parent to Tommy (12) and Andrea (3). Her care of the children is erratic and on a number of occasions they have been reported to be at home alone overnight, with no food in the house. Tommy is very protective of his mother and Andrea, but is frequently late for school because he has to 'sort out' things at home.

How can Shelley and her children best be supported by local agencies?

FURTHER READING

DoH (2003) *Every Child Matters*, London, DoH.
The Green Paper on children's services which, in terms of workforce planning issues, looks to the development of interprofessional training for a more cohesive childcare workforce.

SSI (2003) *Modern Social Services: A Commitment to Reform. The 12th Annual Report of the Chief Inspector of Social Services 2002/2003*, London, DoH.
This report draws on a range of inspection and performance review activity of the SSI to provide an assessment of the performance of councils with social services responsibilities across England. The report illustrates regional highlights and provides information about the activities of the SSI.

Bibliography

Abbott, D. Morris, J. and Ward, L. (2001) *The Best Place to be? Policy, Practice and the Experience of Residential School Placements for Disabled Children*, York, Joseph Rowntree Foundation.

Action on Elder Abuse (1996) *The Abuse of Older People at Home, Information for Workers*, London, Action on Elder Abuse.

Adams, A. and Wilson, D. (1996) *Older People with Mental Health Difficulties: User Preferences and Housing Options*, Scotland, Age Concern.

Adams, R. (1998) 'Social work processes', in R. Adams, L. Dominelli and M. Payne (eds) *Social Work, Themes, Issues and Critical Debates*, Basingstoke, Macmillan – now Palgrave Macmillan, pp. 253–72.

ADSS (1991) *Adults at Risk: Guidance for Directors of Social Services*, Stockport, Association of Directors of Social Services.

ADSS (1995) *Mistreatment of Older People: A Discussion Document*, Wolverhampton, Association of Directors of Social Services.

ADSS/LGA (2003) *All Our Tomorrows: Inverting the Triangle of Care. A Joint Discussion Document on the Future of Services for Older People*, London, ADSS.

Advisory Council on the Misuse of Drugs (2003) *Hidden Harm: Responding to the Needs of Children of Problem Drug Users*, London, Home Office.

Age Concern (1994) *The Next Steps: Lessons for the Future of Community Care*, London, Age Concern.

Ahmad, W.I.U. (ed.) (1993) *'Race' and Health in Contemporary Britain*, Buckingham, Open University Press.

Ahmad, W. and Atkin, K. (eds) (1996) *'Race' and Community Care*, Buckingham, Open University Press.

Ahulu, S. (1995) 'Discharge to the community of older patients from hospital', *Nursing Times*, **91**(28).

Alaszewski, A. and Wun, W.-L. (1994) 'Residential services', in N. Malin (ed.) *Implementing Community Care*, Buckingham, Open University Press, pp. 157–73.

Aldridge, J. and Becker, S. (1993) *Children Who Care: Inside the World of Young Carers*, Loughborough University, Department of Social Services.

Allen, K. (2001) *Communication and Consultation, Exploring Ways for Staff to Involve People with Dementia in Developing Services*, York, Joseph Rowntree Foundation/ Policy Press.

Arber, S. and Gilbert, N. (1993) 'Men, the forgotten carers', in J. Walmsley, J. Reynolds, P. Shakespeare and R. Woolfe (eds) *Health, Welfare and Practice. Reflecting on Roles and Relationships*, London, Sage/Open University Press, pp. 107–13.

Arblaster, L. Conway, J. Foreman, A. and Hawtin, M. (1996) *Setting Us Up to Fail? A Study of Inter-agency Working to Address Housing, Health and Social Care Needs of People in General Needs Housing*, Bristol, Policy Press.

Arksey, H. Hepworth, D. and Qureshi, H (2000) *Carers' Needs and the Carers Act*, University of York, Social Policy Research Unit.

Askham, J. and Thompson, C. (1990) *Dementia and Home Care*, London, Age Concern.

Aspsis, S. (2002) 'What they don't tell disabled people with learning difficulties', in M. Corker and S. French (2002) *Disability Discourse*, Buckingham, Open University, pp. 173–82.

Atkin, K. and Rollings, J. (1993) *Community Care in Multi-Racial Britain; a Critical Review of the Literature*, London, Social Policy Research Unit/HMSO.

Atkinson, D. (1986) 'Engaging competent others: A study of the support networks of people with mental handicap', *British Journal of Social Work*, 16, Supplement, pp. 83–101.

Audit Commission (1986) *Making a Reality of Community Care*, London, HMSO.

Audit Commission (2000) *Getting in on the Act: A Review of Progress on Special Educational Needs* (Update) London, Audit Commission.

Audit Commission (2000a) *Forget-Me-Not*, London, Audit Commission.

Audit Commission (2002) *Forget-Me-Not 2002*, London, Audit Commission.

Audit Commission (2002a) *Integrated Services for Older People: Building a Whole Systems Approach in England*, London, Audit Commission.

Audit Commission (2003) *Changing Habits*, London, Audit Commission.

Audit Commission (2004) *Human Rights: Improving Public Service Delivery*, London, Audit Commission.

Avery, D.M. (2002) 'Talking "tragedy", identity issuers in the parental story of disability', in M. Corker and S. French, *Disability Discourse*, Buckingham, Open University, pp. 116–26.

Baldwin, S. and Lunt, N. (1996) *Charging Ahead: The Development of Local Authority Charging Policies for Community Care*, York, Joseph Rowntree Foundation.

Balloch, S. and McLean, J. (2000) 'Human resources in social care', in B. Hudson (ed.) *The Changing Role of Social Care*, London, Jessica Kingsley, pp. 85–102.

Balloch, S. and Taylor, M. (eds) (2001) *Partnership Working, Policy and Practice*, Bristol, Policy Press.

Bamford, T. (1990) *The Future of Social Work*, Basingstoke, Macmillan – now Palgrave Macmillan.

Bamford, T. (2001) *Commissioning and Purchasing*, London, Routledge/Community Care.

Banks, P. (2002) *Partnerships under Pressure. A Commentary on Progress in Partnership-working between the NHS and Local Government*, London, King's Fund.

Banks, P. (2003) *The Struggle for Disability Living Allowance*, Scotland, Disability Agenda.

Banks, S. (2001) *Ethics and Values in Social Work*, 2nd edn, Basingstoke, Palgrave – now Palgrave Macmillan.

Barclay Report (1982) *Social Workers, Their Role and Tasks*, London, Bedford Square Press.

Barnes, C. Oliver, M. and Burton, L. (2002) *Disability Studies Today*, Cambridge, Policy Press.

Barnes, M. and Sullivan, H. (2002) 'Building capacity for collaboration in English health action zones', in C. Glendinning, M. Powell and K. Rummery (eds) *Partnership, New London and the Governance of Welfare*, Bristol, Policy Press.

Barrett, D. (1996) 'Research, theory and practice: misunderstanding verbal language during community care assessments', in J. Phillips and B. Penhale (eds) *Researching Care Management for Older People*, London, Jessica Kingsley.

BASW (2002) *Code of Ethics for Social Work*, London, BASW.

Bateman, N. (2000) *Advocacy Skills for Health and Social Care Professionals*, London, Jessica Kingsley.

Bauld, L. Chesterman, J. and Judge, K. (2000) 'Measuring satisfaction with social care amongst older service users, issues from their literature', *Health and Social Care in the Community*, 18, pp. 316–24.

Bennett, D. and Morris, J. (1983) 'Deinstitutionalisation in the UK', *International Journal of Mental Health*, 2.

Bernard, M. (ed.) (1987) *Developing Services for Elderly Mentally Infirm People: Responses to the 'Rising Tide' Initiative*, Stoke-on-Trent, Beth Johnson Foundation.

Best, D. (1994) *Purchasing and Controlling Skills*, London, CCETSW.

Bewley, C. and Glendinning, C. (1994) *Involving Disabled People in Community Care Planning*, York, Joseph Rowntree Foundation.

Bichard Inquiry Report (2004) HC653, London, Stationery Office.

Biestek, F. (1957) *The Casework Relationship*, London, Unwin.

Bigby, C. (2004) *Ageing with a Lifetime Disability, A Guide to Practice, Program and Policy Issues for Human Services Professionals*, London, Jessica Kingsley.

Biggs, S. (1991) 'Community care, case management and the psychodynamic perspective', *Journal of Social Work Practice*, 5(1) pp. 71–81.

Biggs, S. (1997) 'Social policy as elder abuse', in Decalmer P. and Glendenning F. (eds) *The Mistreatment of Elderly People*, London, Sage, pp. 74–87.

Bion. W.R. (1967) 'Notes on memory and desire', *Psychoanalytic Forum*, 2, pp. 272–3.

Bird, J. and Davies, M. (1996) *Supervision Registers, an Exploratory Study*, Norwich, Social Work Monographs, UEA.

Blackwell, D. (1997) 'Holding, containing and bearing witness: the problem of helpfulness in encounters with torture survivors', *Journal of Social Work Practice*, 11, pp. 81–9.

Bland, R. (ed.) (1996) *Developing Services for Older People and their Families*, London, Jessica Kingsley.

Blyth, E. (2001) 'The impact of the first term of the new Labour government on social work in Britain: the interface between education policy and social work', *British Journal of Social Work*, 31, pp. 563–77.

BMA (1994) *Survey on the Implementation of the Community Care Reforms*, London, BMA.

BMA (2003) *Consent Tool Kit* (available at www.bma.org.uk/ap.nsf/content/consenttk2) (accessed 14.12.04).

BMA/Law Society (2003) *Assessment of Mental Capacity: Guidance for Doctors and Lawyers*, 2nd edn, London, BMA Books.

Bonell, C. (2000) *Into the Mainstream? The Implications for HIV Services of Greater Integration with Sexual and Other Health Services in the UK*, London, DoH.

Booth, T. and Booth, W. (1994) *Parenting under Pressure, Mothers and Fathers with Learning Difficulties*, Buckingham, Open University Press

Bornat, J., Pereira, C., Pilgrim, D. and Williams, F. (eds) (1993) *Community Care: A Reader*, Buckingham, Open University Press

Bradley, G. and Manthorpe, J. (1995) 'The dilemmas of financial assessment, professional and ethical difficulties', *Practice*, 7(4), pp. 21–30.

Bradley, G. and Manthorpe, J. (2000) *Working on the Fault Line*, Birmingham, Venture Press.

Brandon, D. and Towell, N. (1989) *Free to Choose: An Introduction to Service Brokerage*, London, Good Impressions Publishing.

Braye, S. and Preston-Shoot, M. (1995) *Empowering Practice in Social Care*, Buckingham, Open University Press.

British Deaf Association (1996) *Visible Voices*, London, British Deaf Association.

Brown, H. and Turk, V. (1992) 'Defining sexual abuse as it affects adults with learning disabilities, *Mental Handicap*, 20, pp. 44–55.

Brown, L. Tucker, C. and Domokos, T. (2003) 'Evaluating the impact of integrated health and social care teams on older people living in the community', *Health and Social Care in the Community*, 11(2), pp. 85–94.

Bulmer, M. (1987) *The Social Basis of Community Care*, London, Allen & Unwin.

Burgner. T (1996) *The Regulation and Inspection of Social Services*, London, DoH.

Burke, B. and Harrison, P. (2002) 'Anti-oppressive practice', in R. Adams, L. Dominelli and M. Payne (eds) *Social Work, Themes, Issues and Critical Debates*, Basingstoke, Macmillan – now Palgrave Macmillan, pp. 227–35.

Burnard, P. (1989) *Counselling Skills for Health Professionals*, London, Chapman & Hall.

Butler, J. (1993) *Bodies that Matter: On the Discursive Limits of 'Sex'*, London, Routledge.

Cambridge, P., Hayes, L., Knapp, M. with Gould, E. and Fenyo, A. (1994) *Care in the Community Five Years on*, Aldershot, Arena.

Cambridge, P., Carpenter, J., Beecham, J. ,Hallam, A. ,Knapp, M., Forrester-Jones, E. and Tate, A. (2002) 'Twelve years on: the long-term outcomes and costs of deinstitutionalisation and community care for people with learning disabilities', *Tizard Learning Disability Review*, 7(3), pp. 34–42.

Cameron, E. Badger, F. and Evers, H. (1996) 'Ethnicity and care management', in J. Phillips, and B. Penhale (eds) *Reviewing Care Management for Older people*, London, Jessica Kingsley.

Carlisle, J. (1996) *The Housing Needs of Ex-prisoners*, York, Joseph Rowntree Foundation.

Challis, D. (1992) 'Community care of elderly people: bringing together scarcity and choice, needs and costs, *Financial Accountability and Management*, 8(2), pp. 77–95.

Challis, D., Darton, R., Johnson, L., Stone, M. and Traske, D. (1995) *Care Management and Health Care of Older People*, Aldershot, Arena.

Cheetham, J., Fuller, R., McIvor, G. and Petch, A. (1992) *Evaluating Social Work Effectiveness*, Buckingham, Open University Press.

Chetwynd, M. and Ritchie, J. (1996) *The Cost of Care: The Impact of Charging Policy on the Lives of Disabled People*, Bristol, Policy Press.

Chouhan, K. and Lusane, C. (2004) *Black Voluntary and Community Sector Funding, Civic Engagement and Capacity-building*, York, Joseph Rowntree Foundation.

Clark, C. (ed.) (2001) *Adult Day Care Services and Social Inclusion*, London, Jessica Kingsley.

Clark, H., Gough, H. and Macfarlane, A. (2004) *'It Pays Dividends': Direct Payments and Older People*, Bristol, Joseph Rowntree Foundation/Policy Press.

Clarke, S. (2000) *Social Work as Community Development: A Management Model for Social Change*, Aldershot, Ashgate.

Clements, L. (1996) *Community Care and the Law*, London, Local Action Group.

Clements, L. (2004) *Community Care and the Law*, 2nd edn, London, Local Action Group.

Clifford, D.J. (1994) 'Towards anti-oppressive social work method', *Practice*, 6(3).

Collins, J. (1996) *Housing, Support and the Rights of People with Learning Disabilities*, York, Joseph Rowntree Foundation.

Connolly, J. (1996) 'Scaling the wall', *Community Care*, 11–17 July, pp. 26–8.

Cope, C. (2003) *Fulfilling Lives: Inspection of Social Care Services for People with Learning Disabilities*, London, DoH.

Corker, M. and Shakespeare, T. (2002) *Embodying Disability Theory*, London, Continuum.

Coulshed, V. (1991) *Social Work Practice, An Introduction*, 2nd edn, Basingstoke, Macmillan – now Palgrave Macmillan.

Coulshed, V. and Orme, J. (1998) *Social Work Practice: An Introduction*, Basingstoke, Macmillan – now Palgrave Macmillan.

Cowan, D. (1995) 'Community care and homelessness: *R. v Wirral Metropolitan Borough Council, ex parte B*', *Modern Law Review*, 58, pp. 256–61.

Cragg, S. (1996) 'Community care update', *Legal Action*, September, pp. 16–18.

Crawshaw, P. Burton, R. and Giller, K. (2003) 'Health action zones and the problem of community', *Health and Social Care in the Community*, 11(1) pp. 36–44.

Croft, S. and Beresford, P. (1990) *From Paternalism to Participation. Involving People in Social Services*, London, Open Services Project.

CSCI (2004) *Leaving Hospital – The Price of Delays*, London, Commission for Social Care Inspection.

Curtice, L. and Petch, A. (2002) *How Does the Community Care?: Public Attitudes to Community Care in Scotland*, Edinburgh, Scottish Executive.

Dalley, C. (1988) *Ideologies of Caring*, Basingstoke, Macmillan – now Palgrave Macmillan.

Dalrymple, J. and Burke, B. (1995) *Anti-oppressive Practice, Social Care and the Law*, Buckingham, Open University Press.

Darton, R.A. (2004) 'Which types of homes are closing? The characteristics of homes which closed between 1996 and 2001', *Health and Social Care in the Community*, 12(3), pp. 254–64.

Davies, B. and Challis, D. (1986) *Matching Resources to Needs in Community Care: An Evaluated Demonstration of a Long-term Care Model*, Aldershot, Gower.

Davies, M. (1994) *The Essential Social Worker*, 3rd edn, Aldershot, Arena.

Davies, M. (ed.) (1997) *The Blackwell Companion to Social Work*, Oxford, Blackwell.

Davies, M. and Connolly, J. (1995) 'The social worker's role in the hospital, seen through the eyes of other professionals', *Health and Social Care in the Community*, 3(5), pp. 301–9.

Davies, M and Connolly, J. (1995a) 'Hospital social work and discharge planning, an exploratory study in East Anglia', *Health and Social Care in the Community*, 3(6) pp. 363–71.

Dawson, A. and Butler, I. (2003) 'The morally active manager' in J. Henderson and D. Atkinson (eds) *Managing Care in Context*, Open University Press/Routledge, pp. 237–56.

Dawson, C. and McDonald, A. (2000) 'Assessing mental capacity: a checklist for social workers', *Practice*, 12(2), pp. 5–20.

Day, P. Klein, R. and Redmayne, S. (1996) *Why Regulate? Regulating Residential Care for Elderly People*, Bristol, Policy Press.

Decalmer, P. and Glendenning, F. (eds) (1997) *The Mistreatment of Elderly People*, London, Sage.

Derrida, J. (1998) *Monolingualism of the Other*, Stanford, Stanford University Press.

Devore, W. and Schlesinger, E.G. (1991) *Ethnic Sensitive Social Work Practice*, 3rd edn, New York, Macmillan.

DHSS (1980) *Inequalities in Health. Report of a Research Working Group* (the Black Report), London, DHSS.

DHSS/Welsh Office (1971) *Better Services for the Mentally Handicapped*, London, HMSO.

Diba, A. (1996) *Meeting the Cost of Continuing Care, Public Views and Perceptions*, York, Joseph Rowntree Foundation.

Dimond, B. (1997) *Legal Aspects of Care in the Community*, Basingstoke, Macmillan – now Palgrave Macmillan.

Doel, M. and Shardlow, S. (1998) *The New Social Work Practice*, Aldershot, Arena.

DoH (1989) *Working for Patients*, Cm 555, London, HMSO.

DoH (1989a) *The Care of Children: Principles and Practice in Regulations and Guidance*, London, HMSO.

DoH (1989b) *Caring for People: Community Care in the Next Decade and Beyond*, Cm 849, London, HMSO.

DoH (1990) *The Health of the Nation*, London, HMSO.

DoH (1990a) *Community Care in the Next Decade and Beyond: Policy Guidance*, London, HMSO.

DoH (1992) *Committed to Quality: Quality Assurance in Social Services Departments*, London, HMSO.

DoH (1992a) *Social Care for Adults with Learning Disabilities (Mental Handicap)*, London, DoH.

DoH (1993) *Monitoring and Development: Assessment Special Study, A Joint SSI/NMHSE Study of Assessment Procedures in Five Local Authority Areas*, London, DoH.

DoH (1993a) *Diversification and the Independent Residential Care Sector*, London, HMSO.

DoH (1994) *Report of the Inquiry into the Care and Treatment of Christopher Clunis*, London, DoH.

DoH (1994a) *Implementing Caring for People: Community Care for People with HIV and AIDS*, London, DoH.

DoH (1994b) *Implementing Caring for People: Role of the GP and Primary Healthcare Team*, London, DoH.

DoH (1995) *Building Bridges: A Guide to Arrangements for Inter-agency Working for the Care and Protection of Severely Disabled People*, London, DoH.

DoH (1995a) *'F' Factor: Reasons Why Some Older People Choose Residential Care*, London, DoH.

DoH (1995b) *NHS Responsibilities for Meeting Continuing Health Care Needs*, London, DoH.

DoH (1997) *Developing Partnerships in Mental Health*, London, DoH.

DoH (1998) *Modernising Health and Social Services: National Priorities Guidance 1999/00–2001/2*, London, DoH.

DoH (1998a) *Modernising Social Services*, London, DoH.

DoH (1999) *Mental Health National Service Framework*, London, DoH.

DoH (1999a) *Effective Care Co-ordination in Mental Health Services*, London, DoH.

DoH (1999b) *Reform of the Mental Health Act 1983. Proposals for Consultation*, London, DoH.

DoH (1999c) *Better Care, Higher Standards Guidance*, London, DoH.

DoH (2000) *An Organisation with a Memory*, London, DoH.

DoH (2000a) *Framework for the Assessment of Children in Need and their Families*, London, DoH.

DoH (2000b) *Valuing People: A New Strategy for Learning Disability for the 21st Century*, London, Stationery Office.

DoH (2000c) *No Secrets: Guidance on Developing and Implementing Multi-agency Policies and Procedures to Protect Vulnerable Adults from Abuse*, London, DoH.

DoH (2002d) *Listening to People: Consultation on the Reform of Social Services Complaints Procedures*, London, DoH.

DoH (2000e) *Reforming the Mental Health Act*, London, DoH.

DoH (2001) *Shifting the Balance of Power within the NHS, Securing Delivery*, London, DoH.

DoH (2001a) *National Service Framework for Older People*, London, DoH.

DoH (2001b) *The Mental Health Policy Implementation Guide*, London, DoH.

DoH (2001c) *The National Strategy for Sexual Health and HIV*, London, DoH.

DoH (2001d) *The Role and Responsibilities of Caldicott Guardians in Social Care*, London, DoH.

DoH (2001e) *The Journey to Recovery: the Government's Vision for Mental Health Care*, London, DoH.

DoH (2001f) *The Essence of Care: Patient-focused Benchmarking for Health Care Practitioners*, London, DoH.

DoH (2001g) *Reforming the NHS Complaints Procedure – a listening document*, London, DoH.

DoH (2001h) *Carers and Disabled Children Act 2000: Policy and Practice Guidance*, London, DoH.

DoH (2001i) *Fairer Charging Policies for Home Care and Other Non-residential Social Service*, London, DoH.

DoH (2001j) *Continuing Care: NHS and Local Councils' Responsibilities*, London, DoH.

DoH (2001k) *Intermediate Care*, London, DoH.

DoH (2001l) *Social Care for Deafblind Children and Adults*, London, DoH.

DoH (2002) *Learning from Bristol: The Department of Health's Response to the Report of the Public Inquiry into Children's Heart Surgery at Bristol Royal Infirmary 1984–1995*, London, DoH.

DoH (2002a) *Changing Habits*, London, DoH.

DoH (2002b) *Mental Health Policy Implementation Guide: Dual Diagnosis Good Practice Guide*, London, DoH.

DoH (2002c) *Mental Health Policy Guide: Adult Acute Inpatient Care Provision*, London, DoH.

DoH (2002d) *Developing Services for Carers and Families of People with Mental Illness*, London, DoH.

DoH (2002e) *Intermediate Care: Moving Forward*, London, DoH.

DoH (2002f) *Planning with People: Towards Person-centred Approaches. Guidance for Implementation Group*, London, DoH.

DoH (2002g) *Fair Access to Services: Guidance on Eligibility Criteria for Adult Social Care*, London, DoH.

DoH (2003) *Care Homes for Adults (18–65) and Supplementary Standards for Care Homes Accommodation Young People aged 16 and 17: National Minimum Standards*, Care Homes Regulations, London, DoH.

DoH (2003a) *Improving Mental Health Services for Black and Minority Ethnic Communities in England*, London, DoH.

DoH (2003b) *Independence Matters: An Overview of the Performance of Social Care Services for Physically and Sensory Disabled People*, London, DoH.

DoH (2003c) *A Guide to Receiving Direct Payments*, London, DoH.

DoH (2003d) *Introduction to Reimbursement*, London, DoH.

DoH (2003e) *Effective Sexual Health Promotion: A Toolkit for Primary Care Trusts and Others Working in the Field of Good Sexual Health and HIV Prevention*, London, DoH.

DoH (2003f) *Every Child Matters: Change for Children*, London, DoH.

DoH (2003g) *Models of Care for Substance Misuse Treatment*, London, DOH.

DoH (2003h) *Support Grant for Social Services for People with HIV/AIDS Financial Year 2003/4*, London, DoH.

DoH (2004) *Vision and Framework for Adult Social Care*, London, DoH.

DOH (2004a) *The NHS Improvement Plan: Putting People at the Heart of Public Services*, London, Stationery Office.

DoH (2004b) *National Service Framework for Children, Young People and Maternity Services*, London, DoH.

DoH (2004c) *Choosing Health: Making Healthier Choices Easier*, Cm 6374, London, DoH.

DoH (2004d) *Community Care Assessment Directions*, London, DoH.

DoH (2004e) *The Ten Essential Shared Capabilities: A Framework for the Whole of the Mental Health Workforce*, London, DoH.

DoH (2005) *National Service Framework for Long Term Conditions*, London, DoH.

DoH (2005a) *Independence, Well-being and Choice: Our Vision for the Future of Social Care for Adults in England*, London, DoH.

DoH/NAT (2003) *Models of Care for the Treatment of Adult Drug Misusers*, London, DoH.

DoH/SSI (1993) *Inspection of Assessment and Care Management Arrangements in Social Services Departments: Interim Overview Report*, London, DoH.

DoH/SSI (1996) *Growing Up and Moving On: Report of a SSI Project on Transition Services for Disabled Young People*, London, DoH.

DoH/SSI (1998) *They Look After Their Own, Don't They?*, London, DoH.

Dominelli, L. (1998) 'Anti-oppressive practice in context', in R. Adams, M. Payne and L. Dominelli (eds) *Social Work: Themes, Issues and Critical Debates*, Basingstoke, Macmillan – now Palgrave Macmillan, pp. 3–22.

Dominelli, L. (2002) 'Anti-oppressive practice in context', in R. Adams, L. Dominelli and M. Payne (eds) *Social Work: Themes, Issues and Critical Debates*, Basingstoke, Macmillan – now Palgrave Macmillan, pp. 3–17.

Dominelli, L. (2002a) *Anti-Oppressive Social Work: Theory and Practice*, Basingstoke, Palgrave – now Palgrave Macmillan.

Dowling, M. (1998) 'An evaluation of social work practice in relation to poverty issues: Do social workers' attitudes and actions correspond?', in J. Cheetham and M. Kazi (eds) *The Working of Social Work*, London, Jessica Kingsley, pp. 135–50.

Doyal, L. and Gough, I. (1990) *A Theory of Human Need*, Basingstoke, Macmillan – now Palgrave Macmillan.

Driver, S. and Martell, L. (1997) 'New Labour's communitarianisms', *Critical Social Policy*, **17**(2) pp. 27–46.

Egan, G. (1990) *The Skilled Helper*, 4th edn, Pacific Grove, CA, Brooks/Cole.

Ellis, K. (1993) *Squaring the Circle: User and Carer Participation in Needs Assessment and Community Care*, University of Birmingham, Joseph Rowntree Foundation.

Evans, T. and Harris, J. (2004) 'Street-level bureaucracy, social work and the (exagerrated) death of discretion', *British Journal of Social Work*, **34**(6), pp. 871–95.

Evercare (2004) *Implementing the Evercare Programme: Interim Report*, London, NHS Modernisation Agency.

Fillit, H., Howe, J.L., Fulop, G., Sach, C. ,Sell, L., Siegel, P., Miller, M. and Butler, R.N. (1992) 'Hospital social stays in the frail elderly and their relationship to the intensity of social work intervention', *Social Work in Health Care*, **18**(1), pp. 1–22.

Finch, J. (1989) *Kinship Obligations and Social Change*, Cambridge, Policy Press.

Finch, J. and Mason, J. (1993) *Negotiating Family Responsibilities*, London, Routledge.

Finkelstein, V. (1993) 'Disability: a social challenge or an administrative responsibility', in J. Swain, V. Finkelstein, S. French and M. Oliver (eds) *Disabling Barriers – Enabling Environments*, London, Sage.

Fisher, M. (1990) 'Care management and social work: clients with dementia', *Practice*, 4(4) pp. 229–41.

Fook, J. (2002) *Social Work: Critical Theory and Practice*, London, Sage.

Fruin, D. (2000) *New Directions for Independent Living, Inspection of Independent Living Arrangements for Younger Disabled People*, London, DoH.

Giller, H. and Tutt, N. (1995) 'Pass the parcel', *Community Care*, 18–24 May.

Glasby, J. (2003) *Hospital Discharge: Integrating Health and Social Care*, Oxford, Radcliffe Medical Press.

Glasby, J. and Littlechild, R. (2004) *The Health and Social Care Divide: The Experiences of Older People*, Bristol, Policy Press.

Goldberg, E.M. and Warburton, R.W. (1979) *Ends and Means in Social Work*, London, George Allen & Unwin.

Goldsmith, M. (1996) *Hearing the Voice of People with Dementia*, London, Jessica Kingsley.

Goodwin, S. (1989) 'Community care for the mentally ill in England and Wales, myths, assumptions and reality', *Journal of Social Policy*, 18, part 1, pp. 27–52.

Gorman, H. and Postle, K. (2003) *Transforming Community Care: A Distorted Vision?*, London, BASW.

Goudie, F. and Alcott, D. (1994) 'Perspectives in training, assessment and intervention', in M. Eastman (ed.) *Old Age Abuse: A New Perspective*, 2nd edn, London, Chapman & Hall.

Grant, G. (2001) 'Older people with learning disabilities: health, community inclusion and family care giving', in M. Nolan, S. Davies and G Grant (eds) *Working with Older People and their Families: Key Issues in Policy and Practice*, Buckingham, Open University Press.

Griffiths, S. (1997) *Housing Benefit and Supported Housing: The Impact of Recent Changes*, York, Joseph Rowntree Foundation.

Griffiths, S. (2000) *Supporting People All the Way: An Overview of the Supporting People Programme*, York, Joseph Rowntree Foundation.

Griffiths, Sir Roy (1988) *Community Care: Agenda for Action*, London, HMSO.

GSCC (2002) *Code of Practice for Social Care Workers*, London, General Social Care Council.

Guest, M. (2002) 'The single assessment', *Professional Social Work*, January, pp. 16–17.

Guillemard, A.-M. (1993) *Old Age and the Welfare State*, London, Sage.

Hadley, R. and McGrath, M. (1984) *When Services are Local – The Normanton Experience*, London, Allen & Unwin.

Hallet, C. and Birchall, E. (1992) *Co-ordination in Child Protection*, London, HMSO.

Hancock, R. (1998) *Can Housing Wealth Alleviate Poverty Among Britain's Older Population?*, Bristol, Fiscal Studies Institute.

Harden, J. (1992) *The Contracting State*, Buckingham, Open University Press.

Harding, T. and Beresford, P. (1996) *The Standards We Expect: What Service Users and Carers Want from Social Services Workers*, London, NISW.

Hasler, F. and Stewart, A. (2004) *Making Direct Payments Work: Identifying and Overcoming Barriers to Implementation*, Brighton, Pavilion/Joseph Rowntree Foundation.

Hayes, D, and Humphries, B. (2004) *Social Work, Immigration and Asylum*, London, Jessica Kingsley.

Health Advisory Service (1983) *The 'Rising Tide', Developing Services for Mental Illness in Old Age*, London, HMSO.

Henwood, M. and Waddington, E. (2002) *Outcomes of Social Care for Adults: Message for Policy and Practice*, Leeds, Nuffield Institute for Health.

Henwood, M. Hardy, B. Hudson, B. and Williams, G. (1997) *Interagency Collaboration, Hospital Discharge and Continuing Care Sub-study*, Leeds, Nuffield Institute for Health.

Heslop, P., Mallett, R., Simons, K. and Ward, L. (2001) *Bridging the Divide: The Experiences of Young People with Learning Difficulties and their Families at Transition*, Norah Fry Research Centre, University of Bristol.

Heywood, F. and Smart, G. (1996) *Trends in Funding Adaptations*, Bristol, Policy Press.

Higgins, J. (1989) 'Defining community care, realities and myths', *Social Policy and Administration*, 23(1), pp. 3–16.

Hirschman, A. (1970) *Exit, Voice and Loyalty: Responses to Decline in Firms, Organisations and States*, Harvard University Press.

Hirst, M. and Baldwin, S. (1994) *Unequal Opportunities: Growing Up Disabled*, London, HMSO.

Hoggett, B. (1989) 'The elderly mentally infirm, procedures for civil commitment and guardianship', in J. Eekalaar and D. Pearl (eds) *An Ageing World*, Oxford, Clarendon Press., pp. 517–30.

Holliday, I. (1995) *The NHS Transformed. A Guide to the Health Reforms*, Manchester, Baseline Books.

Holman, A. with Bewley, C. (2000) *Funding Freedom 2000: People with Learning Difficulties using Direct Payments*, London, Values into Action.

Home Office (1995) *Making a Difference*, London, HMSO.

Homer, A.C. and Gilleard, C. (1990) 'Abuse of elderly people by their carers', *British Medical Journal*, 301, pp. 1359–62.

Horne, M. (1999) *Values in Social Work*, Aldershot, Ashgate.

Horwath, J. (2003) 'Child care practice: inspections for assessments across specialisms', in J. Horwath and S. Shardlow (eds) *Making Links across Specialisms. Understanding Modern Social Work Practice*, Lyme Regis, Russell House.

House of Commons Health Committee (1996) *Long Term Care, Future Provision and Funding*. Third Report. Vol. 1, HC 59–61, London, Stationery Office.

House of Commons Health Committee (2002) *Delayed Discharges*. Third Report, HC 617-I, London, Stationery Office.

Howe, D. (1994) 'Modernity, postmodernity and social work', *British Journal of Social Work*, 24(5), pp. 513–32.

Howe, D. (1996) Values in Social Work, personal communication.

Hoyes, L., Jeffers, S., Lart, T., Means, R. and Taylor, M. (1993) *User Empowerment and the Reform of Community Care*, Bristol, School of Advance Urban Studies.

Hudson, J. Watson, L. and Allan, G. (1996) *Moving Obstacles, Housing Choices and Community Care*, Bristol, Policy Press.

Hughes, B. (1993) 'A model for the comprehensive assessment of older people and the carers', *British Journal of Social Work*, 23, pp. 345–64.

Hughes, B. (1995) *Older People and Community Care*, Buckingham, Open University Press.

Humphrey, J. (2003) 'New Labour and the regulatory reform of social care', *Critical Social Policy*, 23(1), pp. 5–24.

Huxley, P. (1990) *Effective Community Mental Health Services*, London, Avebury.

Huxley, P. (1993) 'Care management and care management in community care', *British Journal of Social Work* 23, pp. 365–81.

IASSW (2001) *International Definition of Social Work*, International Association of Schools of Social Work at www.iassw.soton.ac.uk.

Jack, R. (1995) *Empowering in Community Care*, London, Chapman & Hall.

Jack, R. (ed.) (1998) *Residential versus Community Care*, Basingstoke, Macmillan – now Palgrave Macmillan.

Jones, K. (1993) *Asylums and After*, London, Athlone Press.

Jones, S. and Joss, R. (1995) 'Models of professionalism', in M. Yelloly and M. Henkel (eds) *Learning and Teaching in Social Work: Towards Reflective Practice*, London, Jessica Kingsley.

Jordan, B. (1995) 'Are the New Right policies sustainable? "Back to basics" and public choice', *Journal of Social Policy*, 24(3) pp. 363–84.

Jordan, B. (1996) *A Theory of Poverty and Social Exclusion*, Cambridge, Policy Press.

Jordan, B. (1997) 'Social work and society', in M. Davies (ed.) *The Blackwell Companion to Social Work*, Oxford, Blackwell, pp. 8–23.

Jordan, B. with Jordan, C. (2000) *Social Work and the Third Way: Tough Love as Social Policy*, London, Sage.

Joseph Rowntree Foundation Inquiry (1996) *Meeting the Costs of Community Care*, York, Joseph Rowntree Foundation.

Kemshall, H. (2002) *Risk, Social Policy and Welfare*, Buckingham, Open University Press.

Kemshall, H. Parton, N. Walsh, M. and Waterson, J. (1997) 'Concepts of risk in relation to organisational structure and functioning within the personal social services and probation', *Social Policy and Administration*, 31(3) pp. 213–32.

Kestenbaum, A. (1993) *Taking Care in the Market: A Study of Agency Homecare*, London, RADAR/DIG.

Kestenbaum, A. (1996) *Independent Living: A Review*, York, Joseph Rowntree Foundation.

Kharicha, K. Levin, E. Iliffe, S. and Davey, B. (2004) 'Social work, general practice and evidence-based policy in the collaborative care of older people, current problems and future possibilities', *Health and Social Care in the Community*, 12(2), pp. 134–41.

Kohli, R. and Mather, R. (2003) 'Promoting psychosocial well-being in unaccompanied asylum seeking young people in the United Kingdom', *Child and Family Social Work*, 8, pp. 201–12.

Laing, W. (2003) *Care of Elderly People Market Survey*, London, Laing & Buisson.

Lamb, B. and Layzell, S. (1995) *Disabled in Britain, Counting on Community Care*, London, SCOPE.

Laming, Lord (2003) *The Victoria Climbié Inquiry. Summary and Recommendations*, London, Stationery Office.

Langan, J. and Means, R. (1994) *Money Matters in Later Life: Financial Management and Elderly People in Kirklees*, Oxford, Anchor Housing Association.

Langan, J. and Means, R. (1996) 'Financial management and elderly people with dementia in the UK', *Ageing in Society*, 16(3), pp. 287–315.

Lapsley, I. (1996) *Market and Choices: Contracts for Care*, ESRC Library and Information Service.

Lapsley, I., Llewellyn, S. and Mitchell, F. (1994) *Cost Management in the Public Sector*, London, Longman.

Law Commission (1995) *Mental Incapacity, Summary of Recommendations, Consultation Paper No. 231*, London, HMSO.

Le Grand, J. and Bartlett, W. (eds) (1993) *Quasi-Markets and Social Policy*, Basingstoke, Macmillan – now Palgrave Macmillan.

Letts, P. (1998) *Managing Other People's Money*, 2nd edn, London, Age Concern.

Levin, E., Sinclair, I. and Gorbach, P. (1989) *Families, Service and Confusion in Old Age*, Aldershot, Gower.

Lewis, J. and Glennerster, H. (1996) *Implementing the New Community Care*, Buckingham, Open University Press.

Lipsky, M (1980) *Street Level Bureaucracy*, New York, Russell Sage.

Lovelock, R. and Powell, J. with Craggs, S. (1995) *Assessing the Social Support Needs of Visually Impaired People*, York, Joseph Rowntree Foundation.

Lymbery, M. (1998) 'Care management and professional autonomy, the impact of community care legislation on social work with older people', *British Journal of Social Work*, 28(6), pp. 863–78.

Lymbery, M. and Millward, A. (2000) 'The primary health care interface', in G. Bradley, and J. Manthorpe (eds) *Working on the Fault Line*, Birmingham, Venture Press, pp. 11–44.

Lyons, K., LaValle, I. and Grimwood, C. (1995) 'Career patterns of qualified social workers; discussion of a recent survey', *British Journal of Social Work*, 25, pp. 173–90.

McCreadie, C. (1996) *Elder Abuse, Update on Research*, London, Age Concern.

McDonald, A. (1993) 'Elder abuse and neglect – the legal framework', *Journal of Elder Abuse and Neglect*, 5(2), pp. 81–96.

McDonald, A. (1997) *Challenging Local Authority Decisions*, Birmingham, Venture Press.

McDonald, A. (2001) 'The Human Rights Act and social work practice', *Practice*, **13**(3), pp. 5–16.

McDonald, A. (2004) *Community Care Law File*, 2nd edn, Norwich, Social Work Monographs, UEA.

McDonald, A. and Taylor, M. (1994) 'Access to health care services and information in residential care', *Journal of Care and Practice*, **3**(4), pp. 41–52.

McDonald, A. and Taylor, M. (1995) *The Law and the Elderly*, London, Sweet & Maxwell.

Macdonald, C. and Myers, F. (1995) *Assessment and Care Management: The Practitioner Speaks*, University of Stirling, Social Work Research Centre.

Macdonald, S. (1991) *All Equal under the Act?* London, REU/NISW.

Mackintosh, S., Means, R. and Leather, P. (1990) *Housing in Later Life*, School of Advanced Urban Studies Study 4, Bristol, School of Advanced Urban Studies.

McLeod, E. (1996) *Working for Equality in Health*, London, Routledge.

McLeod, E., Bywaters, P. and Cooke, M. (2003) 'Social work in accident and emergency departments: a better deal for older patients' health', *British Journal of Social Work*, **33**, pp. 787–802.

Macpherson Report (1999) *The Stephen Lawrence Inquiry*, Cm 4262–1, London, Stationery Office.

McPherson, B. (1988) 'Whose best interests?', *Social Work Today*, 22 September.

McWilliams, C.L., Brown, J.B., Carmichael, J.L. and Lehman, J.M. (1994) 'A new perspective on threatened autonomy in elderly persons – the disempowering process', *Social Science and Medicine*, **38**(2), pp. 327–38.

Malin, N. (ed.) (1994) *Implementing Community Care*, Buckingham, Open University Press.

Malin, N., Wilmot, S. and Manthorpe, J. (2002) *Key Concepts and Debates in Health and Social Policy*, Buckingham, Open University Press.

Malpas, P. and Means, R. (eds) (1993) *Implementing Housing Policy*, Milton Keynes, Open University Press.

Mandelstam, M. (1997) *Equipment for Older or Disabled People and the Law*, London, Jessica Kingsley.

Marks, L. (1994) *Seamless Care or Patchwork Quilt? Discharging Patients from Acute Hospital Care*, London, King's Fund.

Marsh, P. (1996) *Business Skills for Care Management: A Guide to Costing, Contracting and Negotiating*, London, Age Concern.

Marsh, P. and Fisher, M. (1992) *Good Intentions: Developing Partnership in Social Services*, York, Joseph Rowntree Foundation.

Martin, G.P., Peet, S.M., Hewitt, G.J. and Parker, H. (2004) 'Diversity in intermediate care', *Health and Social Care in the Community*, **12**(2) pp. 150–4.

Mattingley, R. (2002) *Supporting People with Multiple Impairments*, York, Joseph Rowntree Foundation.

Mattison, J. and Sinclair, I. (1979) *Mate and Stalemate*, London, Institute of Marital Studies.

Mayo, J. (1994) *Communities and Caring: The Mixed Economy of Welfare*, New York, St. Martin's Press.

Means, M. (1997) 'Housing options in 2020, a suitable home for all?' in M. Evandrou (ed.) *Baby Boomers, Ageing in the 21st Century*, London, Age Concern, pp. 142–64.

Means, R. and Smith, R. (1994) *Community Care, Policy and Practice*, Basingstoke, Macmillan – now Palgrave Macmillan.

Means, R., Morbey, H. and Smith, R. (2002) *From Community Care to Market Care?: The Development of Welfare Services for Older People*, Bristol, Policy Press.

Medical Foundation for AIDS and Sexual Health (2003) *Recommended Standards for NHS HIV Services*, London, DoH.

Mencap (1995) *Community Care, Britain's Other Lottery*, London, Mencap.

MIND (2002) *Roads to Recovery*, London, MIND.

Moriarty, J. and Webb, S. (1997) *Part of their Lives: An Evaluation of Community Care Arrangements for Older People with Dementia*, London, NISW.

Morris, J. (1993) 'Us and them? Feminist research and community care', in J. Bornat, C. Pereira, D. Pilgrim and F. Williams (eds) *Community Care: A Reader*. Buckingham, Open University Press, pp. 160–7.

Morris, J. (1994) 'Community care or independent living?', *Critical Social Policy*, 40, pp, 25–45.

Morris, J. (2003) *Young Disabled People Moving into Adulthood*, York, Joseph Rowntree Foundation.

Mountain, G. and Pighills, A. (2003) 'Pre-discharge home visits with older people, time to review practice', *Health and Social Care in the Community*, 11(2), pp. 146–54.

NACRO (1996) *Keeping Your Home: Information for Prisoners on Getting Housing Costs Paid*, London, NACRO.

National Institute of Adult Continuing Education (1996) *Still a Chance to Learn?*, Leicester, NIACE.

Neill, J. and Williams, J. (1992) *Leaving Hospital: Elderly People and their Discharge to Community Care*, London, HMSO.

Neill, J., Sinclair, I., Gorbach, P. and Williams, J. (1988) *A Need for Care? Elderly Applicants for Local Authority Homes*, Aldershot, Avebury.

New, B. and LeGrand, J. (1996) *Rationing in the NHS: Principles and Pragmatism*, London, King's Fund.

NIMHE (2003) *Inside Outside: Improving Mental Health Services for Black and Minority Ethnic Communities in England*, London, NIMHE.

NIMHE (2004) *Scoping Review on Mental Health Anti-Stigma and Discrimination*, London, NIMHE.

Nocon, A. and Baldwin, S. (1998) *Trends in Rehabilitation Policy: A Review of the Literature*, London, King's Fund.

Nocon, A. and Qureshi, H. (1996) *Outcomes of Community Care for Users and Carers: A Social Services Perspective*, Buckingham, Open University Press.

Norman, A. (1980) *Rights and Risks*, London, National Corporation for the Care of Old People.

O'Brien, C.L. and O'Brien, J. (2000) *The Origins of Person-Centred Planning, A Community of Practice Perspective*, Syracuse, Responsive Systems Associates.

O'Brien, J. and Lyle, C. (1987) *Framework for Accomplishment*, Atlanta, Georgia, Responsive Systems Associates.

ODPM (2003) *Supporting People: Policy into Practice*, London, Office of the Deputy Prime Minister.

OGC/Home Office (2004) *Think Smart … Think Voluntary Sector! Good Practice Guidance on Procurement of Services from the Voluntary and Community Sector*, London, Office of Government Commerce/Home Office.

Ogg, J. and Bennett, G. (1992) 'Elder abuse in Britain', *British Medical Journal*, 305, pp. 998–9.

Oldman, C. (2000) *Blurring the Boundaries: A Fresh Look at Housing and Care Provision for Older People*, Brighton, Pavilion.

Oliver, M. (1996) *Understanding Disability: From Theory to Practice*, Basingstoke, Macmillan – now Palgrave Macmillan.

Øvretveit, J. (1993) *Co-ordinating Community Care: Multidisciplinary Teams and Care Management*, Buckingham, Open University Press.

Øvretveit, J., Mathias, P. and Thompson, T. (eds) (1997) *Interprofessional Working for Health and Social Care*, Basingstoke, Macmillan – now Palgrave Macmillan.

Parker, G. (1993) *With This Body: Caring and Disability in Marriage*, Buckingham, Open University Press.

Parton, N., Thorpe, D.H. and Watson, C. (1997) *Child Protection: Risk and the Moral Order*, Basingstoke, Macmillan.

Patmore, C. (2001) 'Can managers research their own services? An experiment in consulting frail, older community care clients', *Managing Community Care*, 9(5), pp. 8–17.

Payne, M. (1995) *Social Work and Community Care*, Basingstoke, Macmillan – now Palgrave Macmillan.

Payne, M. (2000) *Teamwork in Multiprofessional Care*, Basingstoke, Macmillan – now Palgrave Macmillan.

Payne, M. (2002) 'Social work theories and reflective practice', in R. Adams, L. Dominelli and M. Payne (eds) *Social Work: Themes, Issues and Critical Debates*, Basingstoke, Macmillan – now Palgrave Macmillan, pp. 123–37.

Peace, S., Kellaher, N. and Willcocks, D. (1997) *Re-evaluating Residential Care*, Buckingham, Open University Press.

Petch, A. (1994) *Assessment and Care Management in Scotland: An Overview*, University of Stirling, Social Work Research Centre.

Petch, A. (1996) *Delivering Community Care: Initial Implementation of Care Management in Scotland*, Edinburgh, Stationery Office.

Petch, A. (2003) *Intermediate Care: What do we Know about Older People's Experiences?*, York, Joseph Rowntree Foundation.

Peters, M. (1998) *Naming the Multiple: Poststructuralism and Education*, London, Bergin and Garvey.

Pfeffer, N. and Coote, A. (1991) *Is Quality Good for You?*, Social Policy Paper no. 5, London, Institute of Public Policy Research.

Phillips, J. (1996) 'Reviewing the literature on care management', in J. Phillips and B. Penhale (eds) *Reviewing Care Management for Older People*, London, Jessica Kingsley.

Phillips, J., Bernard, M. and Chittenden, M. (2002) *The Experiences of Working Carers of Older-adults*, York, Joseph Rowntree Foundation.

Pietroni, M. (1995) 'The nature and aims of professional education for social workers, a post-modern perspective', in M. Yelloly and M. Henkel (eds) *Learning and Teaching in Social Work: Towards Reflective Practice*, London, Jessica Kingsley.

Pilling, D. (1992) *Approaches to Community Care for People with Disabilities*, London, Jessica Kingsley.

Pinfold, V., Hoxley, P., Thornicroft, G. et al. (2003) 'Reducing psychiatric stigma and discrimination: evaluating an educational intervention with the police force in England', *Social Psychiatry and Psychiatric Epidemiology*, 38(6), pp. 337–44.

Postle, K. (2001) 'The social work side is disappearing. I guess it started with us being called care managers', *Practice*, 13(1), pp. 13–26.

Postle, K. (2002) 'Working "between the idea and the reality", ambiguities and tensions in care managers' work', *British Journal of Social Work*, 32(3), pp. 335–52.

Poxton, R. (2003) 'What makes effective partnership between health and social care?', in J. Glasby and E. Peck (eds) *Care Trusts: Partnership Working in Action*, Oxford, Radcliffe Medical Press.

Preston-Shoot, M. and Wigley, V. (2002) 'Closing the circle, social workers' responses to multi-agency procedures on older age abuse', *British Journal of Social Work*, 32, pp. 299–320.

Price Waterhouse/DoH (1991) *Implementing Community Care: Purchaser, Commissioner and Provider Roles*, London, HMSO.

Price, J. and Shildrick, M. (2002) 'Bodies together, touch, ethics and disability', in M. Corker and T. Shakespeare (eds) *Embodying Disability Theory*, London, Continuum, pp. 62–75.

Priestley, M. (1998) *Disability Politics and Community Care*, London, Jessica Kingsley.

Priestley, M. (2000) 'Adults only, disability, social policy and the life course', *Journal of Social Policy*, **29**(3), pp. 421–39.

Priestley, M. (2003) *Disability: A Life Course Approach*, Cambridge, Policy Press.

Prime Minister's Strategy Unit (2004) *Improving the Life Chances of Disabled People*, London, Cabinet Office.

Pritchard, J. (2000) *The Needs of Older Women: Services for Victims of Elder Abuse and Other Abuse*, Bristol, Policy Press.

PSSRU (1996) *Bulletin*, University of Kent, Personal Social Services Research Unit.

QAA (2000) *Social Policy and Administration and Social Work: Subject Benchmark*, London, Quality Assurance Agency for Higher Education.

Quilgars, D. (2004) *Community Care Development: A New Concept*, York, Joseph Rowntree Foundation.

Qureshi, H., Challis, D.J. and Davies, B.P. (1983) 'Motivation and reward of helpers in the Kent Community Care Scheme', in S. Hatch (ed.) *Volunteers, Patterns, Meaning and Motives*, Berkhamstead, The Volunteer Centre.

RADAR (1992) *Disabled People Have Rights*. London, RADAR.

Radia, K. (1996) *Ignored, Silenced, Neglected: Housing and Mental Health Care Needs of Asian People*, York, Joseph Rowntree Foundation.

Raiff, N.R. and Shore, B.K. (1993) *Advanced Case Management: New Strategies for the Nineties*, California, Sage.

Rapp, R.C. (2002) 'Strengths-based case management, enhancing treatment for persons with substance abuse problems', in D. Saleebey (ed.) *The Strengths Perspective in Social Work*, 3rd edn, Boston, MA, Allyn & Bacon.

Ratoff, L. (1973) 'More social work for general practice?', *Journal of the Royal College of General Practitioners*, **23**, pp. 736–42.

Raynes, N., Temple, B., Glenister, C. and Coulthard, L. (2001) *Quality at Home for Older People: Involving Service Users in Defining Home Care Specification*, York, Joseph Rowntree Foundation.

Reed, J. and Stanley, D. (2003) 'Improving communication between hospitals and care homes, the development of a daily living plan for older people', *Health and Social Care in the Community*, **11**(4), pp. 356–63.

Rees, S. (1991) *Achieving Power: Practice and Policy in Social Welfare*, North Sydney, Allen & Unwin.

Refugee Council (2004) *Hungry and Homeless: The Impact of the Withdrawal of State Support on Asylum Seekers*, London, Refugee Council.

Reigate, N. (1995) *The Social Worker as Care Manager*, Norwich, Social Work Monographs, UEA.

Reigate, N. (1997) 'Networking', in M. Davies (ed.) *The Blackwell Companion to Social Work*, Oxford, Blackwell, pp. 214–22.

Renshaw, J. (1988) 'Care in the community, individual care planning and case management', *British Journal of Social Work*, **18** (Supplement), pp. 79–105.

Richards, S. (2000) 'Bridging the divide, elders and the assessment process', *British Journal of Social Work*, **30**, pp. 37–49.

Robertson, S. (1995) *Fed and Watered: The Views of Older People on Need, Assessment and Care Management*, Age Concern, Scotland.

Robinson, C. and Williams, V. (2002) 'Carers of people with learning disabilities, and the experience of the 1995 Carers Act', *British Journal of Social Work* **32**, pp. 169–83.

Rogers, C. (1967) *On Becoming a Person: A Therapist's View of Psychotherapy*, London, Constable.

Royal Commission on Long Term Care (1999) *With Respect to Old Age: Long Term Care – Rights and Responsibilities*, London, Stationery Office.

Royal Commission on Long Term Care (2003) *Long-term Care, Statement by Royal Commissioners*, London, Stationery Office.

Rummery, K. (2002) *Disability, Citizenship and Community Care: A Case for Welfare Rights?*, Aldershot, Ashgate.

Russell , L. (1995) *Mixed Fortunes: The Funding of the Local Voluntary Sector*, York, Joseph Rowntree Foundation.

Sainsbury Centre for Mental Health (2002) *Breaking the Circles of Fear: A Review of the Relationship between Mental Health Services and African and Caribbean Communities*, London, Sainsbury Centre.

Sainsbury, E. (1975) *Social Work with Families*, London, Routledge & Kegan Paul.

Sale, A. (2003) 'Social services staff to play a major role in schools offering new services', *Community Care*, April 24–30, pp. 14–15.

Saleebey, D. (ed.) (2002) *The Strengths Perspective in Social Work Practice*, 3rd edn, Boston, MA, Allyn & Bacon.

Schön, D. (1993) *The Reflective Practitioner*, New York, Basic Books.

SCIE (2004) *Has Service User Participation Made a Difference to Social Care Services?*, London, SCIE.

Scottish Executive (2000) *Community Care: A Joint Future*, Edinburgh, Scottish Executive.

Scottish Executive (2001) *Response to the Report of the Joint Future Group*, Edinburgh, Scottish Executive.

Seed, P. (1988) *Day Care at the Crossroads*, Tunbridge Wells, Costello.

Seed, P. (1990) *Introducing Network Analysis in Social Work*, London, Jessica Kingsley.

SFHA (1995) *Medical Priority in Housing Allocation*, Briefing Paper No. 7, Edinburgh, Scottish Federation of Housing Associations.

Shaping our Lives National User Network (2003) *Social Services Users' Own Definitions of Quality Outcomes*, York, Joseph Rowntree Foundation.

Shardlow, S. (2002) 'Values, ethics and social work', in R. Adams, L. Dominelli and M. Payne (eds) *Social Work: Themes, Issues and Critical Debates*, 2nd edn, Basingstoke, Macmillan – now Palgrave Macmillan, pp. 30–9.

Sheppard, M. (1995) *Care Management and the New Social Work: A Critical Analysis*, London, Whiting and Birch/SCA (Education).

Simiç, P. (1996) 'What's in a word? From social "worker" to care "manager"', *Practice*, 7(3), pp. 5–18.

Sinclair, I., Gibbs, I. and Hicks, L. (2003) *The Management and Effectiveness of the Home Care Service*, York, SWRDU Publications.

Sinclair, I., Parker, R., Leat, D. and Williams, J. (1990) *The Kaleidoscope of Care*, London, HMSO.

Smale, G. and Tuson, G. with Biehal, N. and Marsh, P. (1993) *Empowerment, Assessment: Care Management and the Skilled Worker*, London, NISW/HMSO.

Social Services Committee (1985) *Second Report: Community Care, House of Commons Paper 13-1, Session 1984–5*, London, HMSO.

Specht, H. and Vickery, A. (eds) (1977) *Integrating Social Work Methods*, London, Allen & Unwin.

SSI (1987) *From Home Help to Home Care*, London, DoH.

SSI (1993) *No Longer Afraid: The Safeguard of Elderly People in Domestic Settings: Practice Guidelines*, London, HMSO.

SSI (1993a) *Inspection of Assessment and Care Management Arrangements in Social Services Departments: Interim Overview Report*, London, DoH.

SSI (1993b) *Whose Life is it Anyway? A Report of an Inspection of Services for People with Multiple Impairments*, London, DoH.

SSI (1994) *Substance Misuse: Commissioning Community Care*, London, DoH.

SSI (1995) *Developing Quality Standards for Home Support Services*, London, DoH.

SSI (1995a) *Assessing Older people with Dementia Living in the Community*, London, DoH.

SSI (1996) *Working Alongside Volunteers: Promoting the Role of Volunteers in Community Care*, London, DoH.

SSI (1996a) *Young Carers: Making a Start*, London, DoH.

SSI (1996b) *'Growing Up and Moving On': Report of an SSI Project on Transition Services for Disabled Young People*, London, DoH.

SSI (1996c) *'Growing Up and Moving On': Report of SSI Workshops on Transition Services for Disabled Young People*, London, DoH.

SSI (1997) *Older People with Learning Disabilities*, London, DoH.

SSI (1997a) *A Service on the Edge: Inspection of Services for Deaf and Hard of Hearing People*, London, DoH.

SSI (1998) *They Look After Their Own Don't They? Inspection of Community Care Services for Black and Ethnic Minority Older People*, London, DoH.

SSI (2000) *A Jigsaw of Services: Inspection of Services to Support Disabled Adults in their Parenting Role*, London, DoH.

SSI (2002) *Improving Older People's Services: Policy into Practice*, London, DoH.

SSI (2002a) *Modernising Mental Health Services: Inspection of Mental Health Services*, London, DoH.

SSI (2003) *Modern Social Services: A Commitment to Reform. The 12th Annual Report of the Chief Inspector of Social Services 2002–03*, London, DoH.

SSI/DoH (1991) *Care Management and Assessment: Practitioners' Guide*, London, HMSO.

SSI/DoH (1991a) *Care Management and Assessment: Managers' Guide*, London, HMSO.

SSI/DoH (1996) *Searching for Service: An Inspection of Service Responses made to the Needs of Disabled Young Adults and their Carers*, London, DoH.

Stainton, T. (2002) 'Taking rights structurally: disability rights and social work responses to direct payments', *British Journal of Social Work*, **32**, pp. 751–63.

Stalker, K. (1994) *Implementing Community Care in Scotland: Early Snapshots*, University of Stirling, Social Work Research Centre.

Stalker, K. (ed.) (1996) *Developments in Short-term Care: Breaks and Opportunities*, London, Jessica Kingsley.

Stalker, K. (2003) *Reconceptualising Work with 'Carers': New Directions for Policy and Practice*, London, Jessica Kingsley.

Stalker, K. and Campbell, I. (2002) *Review of Care Management in Scotland*, Edinburgh, Stationery Office.

Stanley, N., Penhale, B., Riordan, D., Barbour, R.S. and Holden, S. (2003) 'Working on the interface: identifying professional responses to families with mental health and child care needs', *Health and Social Care in the Community*, **11**(3) pp. 208–18.

Stevenson, O. (1996) *Elder Protection in the Community: What can we Learn from Child Protection*, London, DoH.

Stevenson, O. and Parsloe, P. (1993) *Community Care and Empowerment*, York, Joseph Rowntree Foundation.

Stewart, G. and Stewart, J. (1993) *Social Work and Housing*, Basingstoke, Macmillan – now Palgrave Macmillan.

Stewart, J. (2000) 'New approaches to local governance', in B. Hudson (ed.) *The Changing Role of Social Care*, London, Jessica Kingsley.

Strauss, A.L. (1964) *Psychiatric Institutions and Ideologies*, New York, Free Press of Glencoe.

Taylor, M., Langan, J. and Hoggett, P. (1995) *Developing Diversity: Voluntary and Private Organisations in Community Care*, Aldershot, Arena.

Thoburn, J. (1986) 'Quality control in child care', *British Journal of Social Work*, **16**, pp. 543–56.

Thoburn, J., Lewis, A. and Shemmings, D. (1995) *Paternalism or Partnership? Family Involvement in the Child Protection Process*, London, HMSO.

Thomas, C. (2002) 'Narrative identity and the disabled self', in M. Corker and S. French (eds) *Disability Discourse*, Buckingham, Open University, pp. 47–55.

Thompson, N. (1993) *Anti-Discriminatory Practice*, Basingstoke, Macmillan – now Palgrave Macmillan.

Thompson, N. (1995) *Age and Dignity: Working with Older People*, Aldershot, Arena.

Thompson, N. (2003) *Promoting Equality: Challenging Discrimination and Oppression*, 2nd edn, Basingstoke, Palgrave – now Palgrave Macmillan.

Thompson, S. and Thompson, N. (1993) *Perspectives on Ageing*, Norwich, Social Work Monographs, UEA.

Tinker, A. (1989) *An Evaluation of Very Sheltered Housing*, London, HMSO.

TOPSS UK (2002) *The National Occupational Standards for Social Work*, London, TOPSS.

Townsend, P. (1981) 'The structural dependency of the elderly, a creation in the twentieth century', *Ageing in Society*, **1**(1) pp. 5–28.

Townsend, P. and Davidson, N. (1992) *Inequalities in Health: the Black Report*, London, Penguin.

Trevithick, P. (2000) *Social Work Skills: A Practice Handbook*, Buckingham, Open University Press.

Turner, M., Brough, P. and Williams-Findlay, R.B. (2003) *Our voice in Our Future: Service Users Debate the Future of the Welfare State*, York, Joseph Rowntree Foundation.

Turner-Crowson, J. and Wallcraft, J. (2002) 'The recovery vision for mental health services and research, a British perspective', *Psychiatric Rehabilitation Journal*, 25(3), pp. 245–54.

Twigg, J. (1989) 'Models of carers: how do social care agencies conceptualise their relationship with informal carers', *Journal of Social Policy*, 18, pp. 53–66.

Valois, N. (2002) 'Maximum discretion!', *Community Care*, 18–24 July, pp. 32–3.

Valois, N. and Sale, A. (2003) 'It's not a race, but . . .', *Community Care*, 10–14 April, pp. 30–3.

Vernon, A. and Qureshi, H. (2000) 'Community care and independence, self-sufficiency or empowerment', *Critical Social Policy*, 20(2), pp. 255–76.

Wagner, G. (1988) *Residential Care. A Positive Choice*, London, HMSO.

Warburton, W. (1989) *Entering Residential Care: A Survey of the Literature*, London, DoH.

Warren, K. (2003) *Exploring the Concept of Recovery from the Perspective of People with Mental Health Problems*, Norwich, Social Work Monographs, UEA.

Watson, L. and Cooper, R. (1992) *Housing with Care*, York, Joseph Rowntree Foundation.

Webb, S. and Levin, E. (2000) 'Locality and hospital-based social work', in G. Bradley and J. Manthorpe (eds) *Working on the Fault Line*, Birmingham, Venture Press, pp. 45–70.

Weinberg, A., Williamson, J., Challis, D. and Hughes, J. (2003) 'What do care managers do? – A study of working practice in older peoples' services', *British Journal of Social Work*, 33, pp. 901–19.

White, L. and Cant, B. (2003) 'Social networks, social support: health and HIV-positive gay men', *Health and Social Care in the Community*, 11(4), pp. 329–34.

Winner, M. (1992) *Quality Work with Older People: Developing Models of Good Practice*, London, CCETSW.

Williams, C. and Evans, J. (2000) *Visible Victims? The Response to Crime and Abuse against People with Learning Disabilities*, Bristol, Joseph Rowntree Foundation.

Willcocks, D., Peace, S. and Kellaher, N. (1987) *Private Lives in Public Places*, London, Tavistock.

Wilson, A. and Beresford, P. (2000) 'Anti-oppressive practice: emancipation or appropriation?', *British Journal of Social Work*, 30, pp. 553–73.

Wilson, A. and Beresford, P. (2002) 'Madness, distress and postmodernity: putting the record straight', in M. Corker and T. Shakespeare (eds) *Embodying Disability Theory*, London, Continuum.

Winchester, R. (2001) 'Up close and personal', *Community Care*, 29 March–4 April 2001, pp. 18–20.

Wistow, G. (1996) 'The changing scene in Britain', in T. Harding, B. Meredith and G. Wistow (eds) *Options for Long term Care: Economic, Social and Ethical Choices*, London, HMSO.

Yelloly, M. and Henkel, M. (1995) *Learning and Teaching in Social Work: Towards Reflective Practice*, London, Jessica Kingsley.

Index